MW00451920

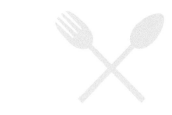

12-WEEK
FOOD JOURNAL &
FITNESS TRACKER

Copyright © 2018 by Rockridge Press, Emeryville, CA.

No part of this publication may be reproduced, stored in a retrieval system, or transmitted in any form or by any means, electronic, mechanical, photocopying, recording, scanning, or otherwise, except as permitted under Section 107 or 108 of the 1976 United States Copyright Act, without the prior written permission of the publisher. Requests to the publisher for permission should be addressed to the Permissions Department, Rockridge Press, 6005 Shellmound Street, Suite 175, Emeryville, CA 94608.

Limit of Liability/Disclaimer of Warranty: The publisher and the author make no representations or warranties with respect to the accuracy or completeness of the contents of this work and specifically disclaim all warranties, including without limitation warranties of fitness for a particular purpose. No warranty may be created or extended by sales or promotional materials. The advice and strategies contained herein may not be suitable for every situation. This work is sold with the understanding that the publisher is not engaged in rendering medical, legal, or other professional advice or services. If professional assistance is required, the services of a competent professional person should be sought. Neither the publisher nor the author shall be liable for damages arising herefrom. The fact that an individual, organization, or website is referred to in this work as a citation and/or potential source of further information does not mean that the author or the publisher endorses the information the individual, organization, or website may provide or recommendations they/it may make. Further, readers should be aware that websites listed in this work may have changed or disappeared between when this work was written and when it is read.

For general information on our other products and services or to obtain technical support, please contact our Customer Care Department within the United States at (866) 744-2665, or outside the United States at (510) 253-0500.

Rockridge Press publishes its books in a variety of electronic and print formats. Some content that appears in print may not be available in electronic books, and vice versa.

TRADEMARKS: Rockridge Press and the Rockridge Press logo are trademarks or registered trademarks of Callisto Media Inc. and/or its affiliates, in the United States and other countries, and may not be used without written permission. All other trademarks are the property of their respective owners. Rockridge Press is not associated with any product or vendor mentioned in this book.

ISBN: 978-1-93975-491-2

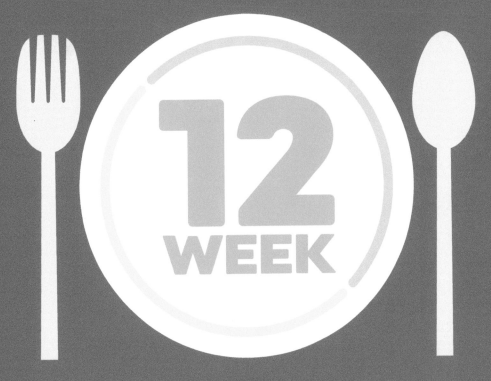

12 WEEK

FOOD JOURNAL &
FITNESS TRACKER

R

ROCKRIDGE
PRESS

The best way to achieve weight loss goals is to hold yourself accountable. With the pages in this journal, you can set your objectives for a 3-month period and plan meals every week with those goals in mind.

GETTING STARTED

My Goals

Date: February 3

1) Lose 10% of my current weight within 3 months.

2) Keep my calorie count to 1200 per day.

3) Eliminate soda and processed foods from my diet.

4) Do at least 30 minutes of cardio every day.

5) Gain more energy and self confidence!

You don't have to focus only on what you want to lose. You can also think about what you want to gain!

> You can fill this in with other nutritional information you'd like to track, such as sodium or cholesterol.

Daily Food Targets

Calories	Carbs	Fat	Protein	Sodium
1200	100g	–	–	1500mg

Daily Lifestyle Targets

Servings of Fruits/Veggies	Cups of Water	Hours of Sleep	Minutes of Exercise
6	11	7.5	30

Starting Stats

	Current	Goal
Weight	205 lbs	185 lbs
Upper Arms	21 in	19 in
Chest		
Waist		
Hips		
Thighs		
Calves		

> List your starting weight and measurements to help you track your progress. Fill in the sections that are important for meeting your goals.

My Plan

Follow a low-carb Mediterranean diet and watch my carbs closely.

Remove soda and processed foods from my pantry and kitchen.

Exercise every day from 8am-9am

Walk or use the treadmill for at least 30 minutes on weekdays.

Bike for 30-60 minutes on the weekends.

Week 1 | Dates: *Feb 3 to Feb 9*

Meal Planner

	Breakfast	Lunch	Dinner	Snacks
MONDAY	Lean bacon	Veggie chili	Chicken gyros	Cantaloupe
	Cantaloupe		Roasted carrots	Baby carrots
	Plain Greek yogurt			

	Breakfast	Lunch	Dinner	Snacks
TUESDAY	Coffee, 1 tsp sugar	Veggie chili	Chicken gyros	Cantaloupe
	1 whole wheat	(leftover)	(leftover)	
	toast		Roasted carrots	

	Breakfast	Lunch	Dinner	Snacks
WEDNESDAY	Lean bacon	Greek salad with	Roasted salmon	Baby carrots
	Cantaloupe	chicken	with quinoa	Cashews
	Plain Greek yogurt		White wine	

	Breakfast	Lunch	Dinner	Snacks
THURSDAY	Coffee, 1 tsp sugar	Greek salad with	Roasted salmon	Baby carrots
	Chocolate-banana	chicken (leftover)	with quinoa	and hummus
	smoothie		(leftover)	

	Breakfast	Lunch	Dinner	Snacks
FRIDAY	Hardboiled egg Chocolate-banana smoothie	Crab cakes with fennel salad	Turkey burger on wheat	Chia pudding

	Breakfast	Lunch	Dinner	Snacks
SATURDAY	Bran muffin Scrambled eggs	White bean soup Apple	Turkey burger on wheat (leftover) Salad greens with Italian dressing	Chia pudding

	Breakfast	Lunch	Dinner	Snacks
SUNDAY	Green juice Scrambled eggs	Greek salad with chicken	Roasted salmon with quinoa White wine	Apple and almond butter Cashews

Notes:

> The meal planning pages will give you a bird's eye view of the week's meals. Planning can help you make healthier choices. You can determine which days you'll have time to cook versus ordering in, and also plan for leftovers for lunch or dinner.

Day 1

Day of the Week | Date: _Monday, Feb 3_

Time: _7:35am_

	Food/Beverage	Calories	Carbs	Fat	Protein	Sodium
BREAKFAST	2 slices lean bacon	30	1	1	4	0
	¼ cantaloupe	46	11	0	1	22
	1 cup plain Greek yogurt	100	6	1	17	61
	Subtotals:	176	18	2	22	83

Time: _10:15am_

	Food/Beverage	Calories	Carbs	Fat	Protein	Sodium
SNACK / SMALL MEAL	½ cup baby carrots	32	6	0	1	64
	Subtotals:	32	6	0	1	64

Time: _12:40pm_

	Food/Beverage	Calories	Carbs	Fat	Protein	Sodium
LUNCH	Veggie chili	343	58	5	19	443
	Subtotals:	343	58	5	19	443

Time: _2:30pm_

	Food/Beverage	Calories	Carbs	Fat	Protein	Sodium
SNACK / SMALL MEAL	¼ cantaloupe	46	11	0	1	22
	Subtotals:	46	11	0	1	22

Time: 7:30pm	Food/Beverage	Calories	Carbs	Fat	Protein	Sodium
DINNER	Chicken gyro w/ tzatziki	289	20	1	50	494
	Roasted carrots	132	17	7	1	235
	Subtotals:	421	37	8	51	729

Time: _____

SNACK / SMALL MEAL

> The diary pages allow you to track what you eat daily as well as maintain your exercise regimen and other healthy habits. You might find that your favorite sandwich is healthier than you thought or that you should drink more water every day.

HOW TO USE
YOUR FOOD
JOURNAL

DAILY TOTALS	Food/Beverage	1018	130	15	94	1341
	Cups of Water	X X X X X X X X X X X ☐ ☐				12
	Cups of Fruits/Veggies	☒ ☒ ☒ ☒ ☐ ☐ ☐ ☐ ☐ ☐ ☐ ☐				5
	Hours of Sleep	X X X X X X ☐ ☐ ☐				7

EXERCISE	Activity	Minutes	Calories Burned
	Brisk walk	40	~150

Notes: Under 1200 calories! But carb totals were a bit high for today, 30g more than target. Adjust portions tomorrow.

Rate how closely you met your goals for today

☐ ☐ ☐ ☐ ☐ ☐ ☐ ☒ ☐ ☐
10% 20% 30% 40% 50% 60% 70% 80% 90% 100%

START YOUR
12 WEEKS

GETTING STARTED

My Goals

Date:

Daily Food Targets

Calories	Carbs	Fat	Protein	

Daily Lifestyle Targets

Servings of Fruits/Veggies	Cups of Water	Hours of Sleep	Minutes of Exercise

Starting Stats

	Current	Goal
Weight		
Upper Arms		
Chest		
Waist		
Hips		
Thighs		
Calves		

My Plan

_____

_____

_____

_____

_____

Week 1 | Dates:

Meal Planner

	Breakfast	Lunch	Dinner	Snacks
MONDAY				
TUESDAY				
WEDNESDAY				
THURSDAY				

	Breakfast	Lunch	Dinner	Snacks
FRIDAY				
SATURDAY				
SUNDAY				

Notes:

Day 1

Time:	Food/Beverage	Calories	Carbs	Fat	Protein	
BREAKFAST	Almond Butter Oatmeal				433	
	Coffee + half+half					
	Subtotals:					

Time:	Food/Beverage	Calories	Carbs	Fat	Protein	
SNACK / SMALL MEAL	+ apple or Suja					
	Subtotals:					

Time:	Food/Beverage	Calories	Carbs	Fat	Protein	
LUNCH	Quinoa Pilaf				487	
	Subtotals:					

Time:	Food/Beverage	Calories	Carbs	Fat	Protein	
SNACK / SMALL MEAL						
	Subtotals:					

Time:	Food/Beverage	Calories	Carbs	Fat	Protein
DINNER	Walnut + Apple Spinach Salad				
	Subtotals:				

Time:	Food/Beverage	Calories	Carbs	Fat	Protein
SNACK / SMALL MEAL	Popcorn				
	Subtotals:				

DAILY TOTALS					
	Food/Beverage				
	Cups of Water	☐☐☐☐☐☐☐☐☐☐☐☐☐☐☐			
	Cups of Fruits/Veggies	☐☐☐☐☐☐☐☐☐☐☐☐			
	Hours of Sleep	☐☐☐☐☐☐☐☐☐☐			

EXERCISE	Activity	Minutes	Calories Burned

Notes:
....
....
....

Rate how closely you met your goals for today

☐ ☐ ☐ ☐ ☐ ☐ ☐ ☐ ☐ ☐
10% 20% 30% 40% 50% 60% 70% 80% 90% 100%

Day 2

Time: ....

	Food/Beverage	Calories	Carbs	Fat	Protein	
BREAKFAST						
	Subtotals:					

Time: ....

	Food/Beverage	Calories	Carbs	Fat	Protein	
SNACK / SMALL MEAL						
	Subtotals:					

Time: ....

	Food/Beverage	Calories	Carbs	Fat	Protein	
LUNCH						
	Subtotals:					

Time: ....

	Food/Beverage	Calories	Carbs	Fat	Protein	
SNACK / SMALL MEAL						
	Subtotals:					

Time: _____	Food/Beverage	Calories	Carbs	Fat	Protein
DINNER					
	Subtotals:				

Time: _____	Food/Beverage	Calories	Carbs	Fat	Protein
SNACK / SMALL MEAL					
	Subtotals:				

DAILY TOTALS					
	Food/Beverage				
	Cups of Water	☐ ☐ ☐ ☐ ☐ ☐ ☐ ☐ ☐ ☐ ☐ ☐ ☐ ☐			
	Cups of Fruits/Veggies	☐ ☐ ☐ ☐ ☐ ☐ ☐ ☐ ☐ ☐ ☐			
	Hours of Sleep	☐ ☐ ☐ ☐ ☐ ☐ ☐ ☐ ☐			

	Activity	Minutes	Calories Burned
EXERCISE			

Notes: _____
_____
_____

Rate how closely you met your goals for today

☐ ☐ ☐ ☐ ☐ ☐ ☐ ☐ ☐ ☐
10% 20% 30% 40% 50% 60% 70% 80% 90% 100%

Day 3

Day of the Week | Date:

Time: _____

	Food/Beverage	Calories	Carbs	Fat	Protein	
BREAKFAST						
	Subtotals:					

Time: _____

	Food/Beverage	Calories	Carbs	Fat	Protein	
SNACK / SMALL MEAL						
	Subtotals:					

Time: _____

	Food/Beverage	Calories	Carbs	Fat	Protein	
LUNCH						
	Subtotals:					

Time: _____

	Food/Beverage	Calories	Carbs	Fat	Protein	
SNACK / SMALL MEAL						
	Subtotals:					

Time: ....

	Food/Beverage	Calories	Carbs	Fat	Protein
DINNER					
	Subtotals:				

Time: ....

	Food/Beverage	Calories	Carbs	Fat	Protein
SNACK / SMALL MEAL					
	Subtotals:				

DAILY TOTALS	Food/Beverage		
	Cups of Water	☐☐☐☐☐☐☐☐☐☐☐☐☐☐	
	Cups of Fruits/Veggies	☐☐☐☐☐☐☐☐☐☐☐	
	Hours of Sleep	☐☐☐☐☐☐☐☐☐	

	Activity	Minutes	Calories Burned
EXERCISE			

Notes: ....

....

....

Rate how closely you met your goals for today

☐ ☐ ☐ ☐ ☐ ☐ ☐ ☐ ☐ ☐
10% 20% 30% 40% 50% 60% 70% 80% 90% 100%

Day 4

Day of the Week | Date:

Time: ....   Food/Beverage   Calories   Carbs   Fat   Protein

BREAKFAST		Calories	Carbs	Fat	Protein
	Subtotals:				

Time: ....

SNACK / SMALL MEAL					
	Subtotals:				

Time: ....

LUNCH					
	Subtotals:				

Time: ....

SNACK / SMALL MEAL					
	Subtotals:				

Time:	Food/Beverage	Calories	Carbs	Fat	Protein
DINNER					
	Subtotals:				

Time:	Food/Beverage	Calories	Carbs	Fat	Protein
SNACK / SMALL MEAL					
	Subtotals:				

DAILY TOTALS						
	Food/Beverage					
	Cups of Water	☐☐☐☐☐☐☐☐☐☐☐☐☐				
	Cups of Fruits/Veggies	☐☐☐☐☐☐☐☐☐☐☐				
	Hours of Sleep	☐☐☐☐☐☐☐☐☐				

EXERCISE	Activity	Minutes	Calories Burned

Notes: ....

Rate how closely you met your goals for today

☐ ☐ ☐ ☐ ☐ ☐ ☐ ☐ ☐ ☐
10% 20% 30% 40% 50% 60% 70% 80% 90% 100%

Day 5

Time: ....

	Food/Beverage	Calories	Carbs	Fat	Protein	
BREAKFAST						
	Subtotals:					

Time: ....

	Food/Beverage	Calories	Carbs	Fat	Protein	
SNACK / SMALL MEAL						
	Subtotals:					

Time: ....

	Food/Beverage	Calories	Carbs	Fat	Protein	
LUNCH						
	Subtotals:					

Time: ....

	Food/Beverage	Calories	Carbs	Fat	Protein	
SNACK / SMALL MEAL						
	Subtotals:					

Time:	Food/Beverage	Calories	Carbs	Fat	Protein
DINNER					
	Subtotals:				

Time:					
SNACK / SMALL MEAL					
	Subtotals:				

DAILY TOTALS	Food/Beverage				
	Cups of Water	☐☐☐☐☐☐☐☐☐☐☐☐☐☐			
	Cups of Fruits/Veggies	☐☐☐☐☐☐☐☐☐☐☐☐			
	Hours of Sleep	☐☐☐☐☐☐☐☐☐			

EXERCISE	Activity	Minutes	Calories Burned

Notes: ....
....
....

Rate how closely you met your goals for today

☐ ☐ ☐ ☐ ☐ ☐ ☐ ☐ ☐ ☐
10% 20% 30% 40% 50% 60% 70% 80% 90% 100%

Day 6

Day of the Week | Date:

Time: _____   Food/Beverage   Calories   Carbs   Fat   Protein

BREAKFAST	Food/Beverage	Calories	Carbs	Fat	Protein
	Subtotals:				

Time: _____

SNACK / SMALL MEAL	Food/Beverage	Calories	Carbs	Fat	Protein
	Subtotals:				

Time: _____

LUNCH	Food/Beverage	Calories	Carbs	Fat	Protein
	Subtotals:				

Time: _____

SNACK / SMALL MEAL	Food/Beverage	Calories	Carbs	Fat	Protein
	Subtotals:				

Time:	Food/Beverage	Calories	Carbs	Fat	Protein
DINNER					
	Subtotals:				

Time:					
SNACK / SMALL MEAL					
	Subtotals:				

DAILY TOTALS	Food/Beverage				
	Cups of Water	☐ ☐ ☐ ☐ ☐ ☐ ☐ ☐ ☐ ☐ ☐ ☐ ☐ ☐			
	Cups of Fruits / Veggies	☐ ☐ ☐ ☐ ☐ ☐ ☐ ☐ ☐ ☐ ☐ ☐			
	Hours of Sleep	☐ ☐ ☐ ☐ ☐ ☐ ☐ ☐ ☐ ☐			

	Activity	Minutes	Calories Burned
EXERCISE			

Notes: ....

....

....

Rate how closely you met your goals for today

☐ ☐ ☐ ☐ ☐ ☐ ☐ ☐ ☐ ☐
10% 20% 30% 40% 50% 60% 70% 80% 90% 100%

Day 7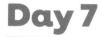

Day of the Week | Date:

Time:	Food/Beverage	Calories	Carbs	Fat	Protein
BREAKFAST					
Subtotals:					

Time:					
SNACK / SMALL MEAL					
Subtotals:					

Time:					
LUNCH					
Subtotals:					

Time:					
SNACK / SMALL MEAL					
Subtotals:					

Time:	Food/Beverage	Calories	Carbs	Fat	Protein
DINNER					
	Subtotals:				

Time:					
SNACK / SMALL MEAL					
	Subtotals:				

DAILY TOTALS	Food/Beverage				
	Cups of Water	☐☐☐☐☐☐☐☐☐☐☐☐☐☐			
	Cups of Fruits/Veggies	☐☐☐☐☐☐☐☐☐☐☐			
	Hours of Sleep	☐☐☐☐☐☐☐☐☐			

	Activity	Minutes	Calories Burned
EXERCISE			

Notes: ....

....

Rate how closely you met your goals for today

☐ ☐ ☐ ☐ ☐ ☐ ☐ ☐ ☐ ☐
10% 20% 30% 40% 50% 60% 70% 80% 90% 100%

Week 2 | Dates:
Meal Planner

	Breakfast	Lunch	Dinner	Snacks
MONDAY				

	Breakfast	Lunch	Dinner	Snacks
TUESDAY				

	Breakfast	Lunch	Dinner	Snacks
WEDNESDAY				

	Breakfast	Lunch	Dinner	Snacks
THURSDAY				

	Breakfast	Lunch	Dinner	Snacks
FRIDAY				
SATURDAY				
SUNDAY				

Notes:

Day 8

Day of the Week | Date:

Time: ....

	Food/Beverage	Calories	Carbs	Fat	Protein
BREAKFAST					
	Subtotals:				

Time: ....

	Food/Beverage	Calories	Carbs	Fat	Protein
SNACK / SMALL MEAL					
	Subtotals:				

Time: ....

	Food/Beverage	Calories	Carbs	Fat	Protein
LUNCH					
	Subtotals:				

Time: ....

	Food/Beverage	Calories	Carbs	Fat	Protein
SNACK / SMALL MEAL					
	Subtotals:				

Time:	Food/Beverage	Calories	Carbs	Fat	Protein
DINNER					
	Subtotals:				

Time:					
SNACK / SMALL MEAL					
	Subtotals:				

DAILY TOTALS	Food/Beverage				
	Cups of Water	☐☐☐☐☐☐☐☐☐☐☐☐☐			
	Cups of Fruits/Veggies	☐☐☐☐☐☐☐☐☐☐☐☐			
	Hours of Sleep	☐☐☐☐☐☐☐☐☐			

	Activity	Minutes	Calories Burned
EXERCISE			

Notes:
....
....
....

Rate how closely you met your goals for today

☐ ☐ ☐ ☐ ☐ ☐ ☐ ☐ ☐ ☐
10% 20% 30% 40% 50% 60% 70% 80% 90% 100%

Day 9

Time: ....

	Food/Beverage	Calories	Carbs	Fat	Protein
BREAKFAST					
	Subtotals:				

Time: ....

		Calories	Carbs	Fat	Protein
SNACK / SMALL MEAL					
	Subtotals:				

Time: ....

		Calories	Carbs	Fat	Protein
LUNCH					
	Subtotals:				

Time: ....

		Calories	Carbs	Fat	Protein
SNACK / SMALL MEAL					
	Subtotals:				

Time:	Food/Beverage	Calories	Carbs	Fat	Protein
DINNER					
	Subtotals:				

Time:					
SNACK / SMALL MEAL					
	Subtotals:				

DAILY TOTALS	Food/Beverage				
	Cups of Water	☐☐☐☐☐☐☐☐☐☐☐☐☐☐			
	Cups of Fruits/Veggies	☐☐☐☐☐☐☐☐☐☐☐			
	Hours of Sleep	☐☐☐☐☐☐☐☐☐			

	Activity	Minutes	Calories Burned
EXERCISE			

Notes: ....
....
....

Rate how closely you met your goals for today

☐ ☐ ☐ ☐ ☐ ☐ ☐ ☐ ☐ ☐
10% 20% 30% 40% 50% 60% 70% 80% 90% 100%

Day 10

Day of the Week | Date:

Time: ....

	Food/Beverage	Calories	Carbs	Fat	Protein
BREAKFAST					
	Subtotals:				

Time: ....

	Food/Beverage	Calories	Carbs	Fat	Protein
SNACK / SMALL MEAL					
	Subtotals:				

Time: ....

	Food/Beverage	Calories	Carbs	Fat	Protein
LUNCH					
	Subtotals:				

Time: ....

	Food/Beverage	Calories	Carbs	Fat	Protein
SNACK / SMALL MEAL					
	Subtotals:				

Time:	Food/Beverage	Calories	Carbs	Fat	Protein
DINNER					
	Subtotals:				

Time:					
SNACK / SMALL MEAL					
	Subtotals:				

DAILY TOTALS	Food/Beverage				
	Cups of Water	☐☐☐☐☐☐☐☐☐☐☐☐☐☐			
	Cups of Fruits/Veggies	☐☐☐☐☐☐☐☐☐☐☐☐			
	Hours of Sleep	☐☐☐☐☐☐☐☐☐			

EXERCISE	Activity	Minutes	Calories Burned

Notes: ....

....

....

Rate how closely you met your goals for today

☐ ☐ ☐ ☐ ☐ ☐ ☐ ☐ ☐ ☐
10% 20% 30% 40% 50% 60% 70% 80% 90% 100%

Day 11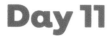

Day of the Week | Date:

Time: _____	Food/Beverage	Calories	Carbs	Fat	Protein
BREAKFAST					
	Subtotals:				

Time: _____					
SNACK / SMALL MEAL					
	Subtotals:				

Time: _____					
LUNCH					
	Subtotals:				

Time: _____					
SNACK / SMALL MEAL					
	Subtotals:				

Time:	Food/Beverage	Calories	Carbs	Fat	Protein
DINNER					
	Subtotals:				

Time:	Food/Beverage	Calories	Carbs	Fat	Protein
SNACK / SMALL MEAL					
	Subtotals:				

DAILY TOTALS					
	Food/Beverage				
	Cups of Water	☐☐☐☐☐☐☐☐☐☐☐☐☐☐☐			
	Cups of Fruits/Veggies	☐☐☐☐☐☐☐☐☐☐☐☐			
	Hours of Sleep	☐☐☐☐☐☐☐☐☐☐			

EXERCISE	Activity	Minutes	Calories Burned

Notes:
....
....
....

Rate how closely you met your goals for today

☐ ☐ ☐ ☐ ☐ ☐ ☐ ☐ ☐ ☐
10% 20% 30% 40% 50% 60% 70% 80% 90% 100%

Day 12

Day of the Week | Date:

Time: ....

	Food/Beverage	Calories	Carbs	Fat	Protein
BREAKFAST					
	Subtotals:				

Time: ....

	Food/Beverage	Calories	Carbs	Fat	Protein
SNACK / SMALL MEAL					
	Subtotals:				

Time: ....

	Food/Beverage	Calories	Carbs	Fat	Protein
LUNCH					
	Subtotals:				

Time: ....

	Food/Beverage	Calories	Carbs	Fat	Protein
SNACK / SMALL MEAL					
	Subtotals:				

Time:	Food/Beverage	Calories	Carbs	Fat	Protein	
DINNER						
	Subtotals:					

Time:						
SNACK / SMALL MEAL						
	Subtotals:					

DAILY TOTALS						
	Food/Beverage					
	Cups of Water	☐ ☐ ☐ ☐ ☐ ☐ ☐ ☐ ☐ ☐ ☐ ☐ ☐ ☐				
	Cups of Fruits/Veggies	☐ ☐ ☐ ☐ ☐ ☐ ☐ ☐ ☐ ☐ ☐ ☐				
	Hours of Sleep	☐ ☐ ☐ ☐ ☐ ☐ ☐ ☐ ☐				

EXERCISE	Activity	Minutes	Calories Burned

Notes: ....
....
....

Rate how closely you met your goals for today

☐ ☐ ☐ ☐ ☐ ☐ ☐ ☐ ☐ ☐
10% 20% 30% 40% 50% 60% 70% 80% 90% 100%

Day 13

Day of the Week | Date:

Time: ....

	Food/Beverage	Calories	Carbs	Fat	Protein
BREAKFAST					
	Subtotals:				

Time: ....

	Food/Beverage	Calories	Carbs	Fat	Protein
SNACK / SMALL MEAL					
	Subtotals:				

Time: ....

	Food/Beverage	Calories	Carbs	Fat	Protein
LUNCH					
	Subtotals:				

Time: ....

	Food/Beverage	Calories	Carbs	Fat	Protein
SNACK / SMALL MEAL					
	Subtotals:				

Time:	Food/Beverage	Calories	Carbs	Fat	Protein
DINNER					
	Subtotals:				

Time:		Calories	Carbs	Fat	Protein
SNACK / SMALL MEAL					
	Subtotals:				

DAILY TOTALS				
	Food/Beverage			
	Cups of Water	☐☐☐☐☐☐☐☐☐☐☐☐☐☐☐		
	Cups of Fruits/Veggies	☐☐☐☐☐☐☐☐☐☐☐☐		
	Hours of Sleep	☐☐☐☐☐☐☐☐☐☐		

EXERCISE	Activity	Minutes	Calories Burned

Notes: ....
....
....

Rate how closely you met your goals for today

☐ ☐ ☐ ☐ ☐ ☐ ☐ ☐ ☐ ☐
10% 20% 30% 40% 50% 60% 70% 80% 90% 100%

Day 14

Day of the Week | Date:

Time: _____

	Food/Beverage	Calories	Carbs	Fat	Protein
BREAKFAST					
	Subtotals:				

Time: _____

	Food/Beverage	Calories	Carbs	Fat	Protein
SNACK / SMALL MEAL					
	Subtotals:				

Time: _____

	Food/Beverage	Calories	Carbs	Fat	Protein
LUNCH					
	Subtotals:				

Time: _____

	Food/Beverage	Calories	Carbs	Fat	Protein
SNACK / SMALL MEAL					
	Subtotals:				

Time:	Food/Beverage	Calories	Carbs	Fat	Protein
DINNER					
	Subtotals:				

Time:					
SNACK / SMALL MEAL					
	Subtotals:				

DAILY TOTALS				
	Food/Beverage			
	Cups of Water	☐☐☐☐☐☐☐☐☐☐☐☐☐☐		
	Cups of Fruits/Veggies	☐☐☐☐☐☐☐☐☐☐☐		
	Hours of Sleep	☐☐☐☐☐☐☐☐☐		

	Activity	Minutes	Calories Burned
EXERCISE			

Notes: ....

....

....

Rate how closely you met your goals for today

☐ ☐ ☐ ☐ ☐ ☐ ☐ ☐ ☐ ☐
10% 20% 30% 40% 50% 60% 70% 80% 90% 100%

Week 3 | Dates:

Meal Planner

	Breakfast	Lunch	Dinner	Snacks
MONDAY				

	Breakfast	Lunch	Dinner	Snacks
TUESDAY				

	Breakfast	Lunch	Dinner	Snacks
WEDNESDAY				

	Breakfast	Lunch	Dinner	Snacks
THURSDAY				

	Breakfast	Lunch	Dinner	Snacks
FRIDAY				
SATURDAY				
SUNDAY				

Notes:

Day 15

Time: _____

	Food/Beverage	Calories	Carbs	Fat	Protein	
BREAKFAST						
	Subtotals:					

Time: _____

	Food/Beverage	Calories	Carbs	Fat	Protein	
SNACK / SMALL MEAL						
	Subtotals:					

Time: _____

	Food/Beverage	Calories	Carbs	Fat	Protein	
LUNCH						
	Subtotals:					

Time: _____

	Food/Beverage	Calories	Carbs	Fat	Protein	
SNACK / SMALL MEAL						
	Subtotals:					

Time:	Food/Beverage	Calories	Carbs	Fat	Protein
DINNER					
	Subtotals:				

Time:					
SNACK / SMALL MEAL					
	Subtotals:				

DAILY TOTALS					
	Food/Beverage				
	Cups of Water	☐☐☐☐☐☐☐☐☐☐☐☐☐☐			
	Cups of Fruits/Veggies	☐☐☐☐☐☐☐☐☐☐☐			
	Hours of Sleep	☐☐☐☐☐☐☐☐☐			

	Activity	Minutes	Calories Burned
EXERCISE			

Notes: ....

....

....

Rate how closely you met your goals for today

☐ ☐ ☐ ☐ ☐ ☐ ☐ ☐ ☐ ☐
10% 20% 30% 40% 50% 60% 70% 80% 90% 100%

Day 16

Day of the Week | Date:

Time: ....

	Food/Beverage	Calories	Carbs	Fat	Protein
BREAKFAST					
	Subtotals:				

Time: ....

	Food/Beverage	Calories	Carbs	Fat	Protein
SNACK / SMALL MEAL					
	Subtotals:				

Time: ....

	Food/Beverage	Calories	Carbs	Fat	Protein
LUNCH					
	Subtotals:				

Time: ....

	Food/Beverage	Calories	Carbs	Fat	Protein
SNACK / SMALL MEAL					
	Subtotals:				

Time:	Food/Beverage	Calories	Carbs	Fat	Protein
DINNER					
	Subtotals:				

Time:		Calories	Carbs	Fat	Protein
SNACK / SMALL MEAL					
	Subtotals:				

DAILY TOTALS					
	Food/Beverage				
	Cups of Water	☐☐☐☐☐☐☐☐☐☐☐☐☐☐			
	Cups of Fruits/Veggies	☐☐☐☐☐☐☐☐☐☐☐☐			
	Hours of Sleep	☐☐☐☐☐☐☐☐☐☐			

EXERCISE	Activity	Minutes	Calories Burned

Notes: ....
....
....

Rate how closely you met your goals for today

☐ ☐ ☐ ☐ ☐ ☐ ☐ ☐ ☐ ☐
10% 20% 30% 40% 50% 60% 70% 80% 90% 100%

Day 17

Day of the Week | Date:

Time: ....

	Food/Beverage	Calories	Carbs	Fat	Protein
BREAKFAST					
	Subtotals:				

Time: ....

	Food/Beverage	Calories	Carbs	Fat	Protein
SNACK / SMALL MEAL					
	Subtotals:				

Time: ....

	Food/Beverage	Calories	Carbs	Fat	Protein
LUNCH					
	Subtotals:				

Time: ....

	Food/Beverage	Calories	Carbs	Fat	Protein
SNACK / SMALL MEAL					
	Subtotals:				

Time:	Food/Beverage	Calories	Carbs	Fat	Protein	
DINNER						
	Subtotals:					

Time:						
SNACK / SMALL MEAL						
	Subtotals:					

DAILY TOTALS						
	Food/Beverage					
	Cups of Water	☐ ☐ ☐ ☐ ☐ ☐ ☐ ☐ ☐ ☐ ☐ ☐				
	Cups of Fruits/Veggies	☐ ☐ ☐ ☐ ☐ ☐ ☐ ☐ ☐ ☐ ☐				
	Hours of Sleep	☐ ☐ ☐ ☐ ☐ ☐ ☐ ☐ ☐				

EXERCISE	Activity	Minutes	Calories Burned

Notes: ....

....

....

Rate how closely you met your goals for today

☐ ☐ ☐ ☐ ☐ ☐ ☐ ☐ ☐ ☐
10% 20% 30% 40% 50% 60% 70% 80% 90% 100%

Day 18

Time: ....

	Food/Beverage	Calories	Carbs	Fat	Protein	
BREAKFAST						
	Subtotals:					

Time: ....

	Food/Beverage	Calories	Carbs	Fat	Protein	
SNACK / SMALL MEAL						
	Subtotals:					

Time: ....

	Food/Beverage	Calories	Carbs	Fat	Protein	
LUNCH						
	Subtotals:					

Time: ....

	Food/Beverage	Calories	Carbs	Fat	Protein	
SNACK / SMALL MEAL						
	Subtotals:					

Time: _____	Food/Beverage	Calories	Carbs	Fat	Protein	
DINNER						
	Subtotals:					

Time: _____	Food/Beverage	Calories	Carbs	Fat	Protein	
SNACK / SMALL MEAL						
	Subtotals:					

DAILY TOTALS						
	Food/Beverage					
	Cups of Water	☐☐☐☐☐☐☐☐☐☐☐☐☐☐				
	Cups of Fruits/Veggies	☐☐☐☐☐☐☐☐☐☐☐☐				
	Hours of Sleep	☐☐☐☐☐☐☐☐☐				

EXERCISE	Activity	Minutes	Calories Burned

Notes: _____

_____

_____

Rate how closely you met your goals for today

☐ ☐ ☐ ☐ ☐ ☐ ☐ ☐ ☐ ☐
10% 20% 30% 40% 50% 60% 70% 80% 90% 100%

Day 19

Time: ....

	Food/Beverage	Calories	Carbs	Fat	Protein
BREAKFAST					
	Subtotals:				

Time: ....

	Food/Beverage	Calories	Carbs	Fat	Protein
SNACK / SMALL MEAL					
	Subtotals:				

Time: ....

	Food/Beverage	Calories	Carbs	Fat	Protein
LUNCH					
	Subtotals:				

Time: ....

	Food/Beverage	Calories	Carbs	Fat	Protein
SNACK / SMALL MEAL					
	Subtotals:				

Time: ....

	Food/Beverage	Calories	Carbs	Fat	Protein
DINNER					
	Subtotals:				

Time: ....

	Food/Beverage	Calories	Carbs	Fat	Protein
SNACK / SMALL MEAL					
	Subtotals:				

DAILY TOTALS	Food/Beverage				
	Cups of Water	☐☐☐☐☐☐☐☐☐☐☐☐☐☐			
	Cups of Fruits/Veggies	☐☐☐☐☐☐☐☐☐☐☐☐			
	Hours of Sleep	☐☐☐☐☐☐☐☐☐			

	Activity	Minutes	Calories Burned
EXERCISE			

Notes: ....

....

....

Rate how closely you met your goals for today

☐ ☐ ☐ ☐ ☐ ☐ ☐ ☐ ☐ ☐
10% 20% 30% 40% 50% 60% 70% 80% 90% 100%

Day 20

Day of the Week | Date:

Time: ....

	Food/Beverage	Calories	Carbs	Fat	Protein
BREAKFAST					
	Subtotals:				

Time: ....

	Food/Beverage	Calories	Carbs	Fat	Protein
SNACK / SMALL MEAL					
	Subtotals:				

Time: ....

	Food/Beverage	Calories	Carbs	Fat	Protein
LUNCH					
	Subtotals:				

Time: ....

	Food/Beverage	Calories	Carbs	Fat	Protein
SNACK / SMALL MEAL					
	Subtotals:				

Time: ....

	Food/Beverage	Calories	Carbs	Fat	Protein
DINNER					
	Subtotals:				

Time: ....

		Calories	Carbs	Fat	Protein
SNACK / SMALL MEAL					
	Subtotals:				

DAILY TOTALS	Food/Beverage				
	Cups of Water	☐☐☐☐☐☐☐☐☐☐☐☐☐☐☐			
	Cups of Fruits / Veggies	☐☐☐☐☐☐☐☐☐☐☐☐			
	Hours of Sleep	☐☐☐☐☐☐☐☐☐☐			

	Activity	Minutes	Calories Burned
EXERCISE			

Notes: ....
....
....

Rate how closely you met your goals for today

☐ ☐ ☐ ☐ ☐ ☐ ☐ ☐ ☐ ☐
10% 20% 30% 40% 50% 60% 70% 80% 90% 100%

Day 21

Day of the Week | Date:

Time: ....

	Food/Beverage	Calories	Carbs	Fat	Protein
BREAKFAST					
	Subtotals:				

Time: ....

	Food/Beverage	Calories	Carbs	Fat	Protein
SNACK / SMALL MEAL					
	Subtotals:				

Time: ....

	Food/Beverage	Calories	Carbs	Fat	Protein
LUNCH					
	Subtotals:				

Time: ....

	Food/Beverage	Calories	Carbs	Fat	Protein
SNACK / SMALL MEAL					
	Subtotals:				

Time:	Food/Beverage	Calories	Carbs	Fat	Protein
DINNER					
	Subtotals:				

Time:					
SNACK / SMALL MEAL					
	Subtotals:				

DAILY TOTALS	Food/Beverage				
	Cups of Water	☐☐☐☐☐☐☐☐☐☐☐☐☐☐			
	Cups of Fruits/Veggies	☐☐☐☐☐☐☐☐☐☐☐☐			
	Hours of Sleep	☐☐☐☐☐☐☐☐☐			

	Activity	Minutes	Calories Burned
EXERCISE			

Notes: ....

....

....

Rate how closely you met your goals for today

☐ ☐ ☐ ☐ ☐ ☐ ☐ ☐ ☐ ☐
10% 20% 30% 40% 50% 60% 70% 80% 90% 100%

Week 4 | Dates:

Meal Planner

	Breakfast	Lunch	Dinner	Snacks
MONDAY				

TUESDAY				

WEDNESDAY				

THURSDAY				

	Breakfast	Lunch	Dinner	Snacks
FRIDAY				
SATURDAY				
SUNDAY				

Notes:

_____

_____

_____

_____

_____

Day 22

Time: ....

	Food/Beverage	Calories	Carbs	Fat	Protein	
BREAKFAST						
	Subtotals:					

Time: ....

	Food/Beverage	Calories	Carbs	Fat	Protein	
SNACK / SMALL MEAL						
	Subtotals:					

Time: ....

	Food/Beverage	Calories	Carbs	Fat	Protein	
LUNCH						
	Subtotals:					

Time: ....

	Food/Beverage	Calories	Carbs	Fat	Protein	
SNACK / SMALL MEAL						
	Subtotals:					

Time:	Food/Beverage	Calories	Carbs	Fat	Protein
DINNER					
	Subtotals:				

Time:					
SNACK / SMALL MEAL					
	Subtotals:				

DAILY TOTALS					
	Food/Beverage				
	Cups of Water	☐☐☐☐☐☐☐☐☐☐☐☐☐			
	Cups of Fruits/Veggies	☐☐☐☐☐☐☐☐☐☐☐			
	Hours of Sleep	☐☐☐☐☐☐☐☐☐			

	Activity	Minutes	Calories Burned
EXERCISE			

Notes:
....
....
....

Rate how closely you met your goals for today

☐ ☐ ☐ ☐ ☐ ☐ ☐ ☐ ☐ ☐
10% 20% 30% 40% 50% 60% 70% 80% 90% 100%

Day 23

Time: ....

	Food/Beverage	Calories	Carbs	Fat	Protein
BREAKFAST					
	Subtotals:				

Time: ....

	Food/Beverage	Calories	Carbs	Fat	Protein
SNACK / SMALL MEAL					
	Subtotals:				

Time: ....

	Food/Beverage	Calories	Carbs	Fat	Protein
LUNCH					
	Subtotals:				

Time: ....

	Food/Beverage	Calories	Carbs	Fat	Protein
SNACK / SMALL MEAL					
	Subtotals:				

Time:	Food/Beverage	Calories	Carbs	Fat	Protein
DINNER					
	Subtotals:				

Time:	Food/Beverage	Calories	Carbs	Fat	Protein
SNACK / SMALL MEAL					
	Subtotals:				

DAILY TOTALS					
	Food/Beverage				
	Cups of Water	☐☐☐☐☐☐☐☐☐☐☐☐☐☐			
	Cups of Fruits/Veggies	☐☐☐☐☐☐☐☐☐☐☐			
	Hours of Sleep	☐☐☐☐☐☐☐☐☐			

EXERCISE	Activity	Minutes	Calories Burned

Notes:

Rate how closely you met your goals for today

☐ ☐ ☐ ☐ ☐ ☐ ☐ ☐ ☐ ☐
10% 20% 30% 40% 50% 60% 70% 80% 90% 100%

Day 24

Day of the Week | Date:

Time: .... Food/Beverage   Calories   Carbs   Fat   Protein

BREAKFAST					
	Subtotals:				

Time: ....

SNACK / SMALL MEAL					
	Subtotals:				

Time: ....

LUNCH					
	Subtotals:				

Time: ....

SNACK / SMALL MEAL					
	Subtotals:				

Time: _____	Food/Beverage	Calories	Carbs	Fat	Protein	
DINNER						
	Subtotals:					

Time: _____	Food/Beverage	Calories	Carbs	Fat	Protein	
SNACK / SMALL MEAL						
	Subtotals:					

DAILY TOTALS					
	Food/Beverage				
	Cups of Water	☐ ☐ ☐ ☐ ☐ ☐ ☐ ☐ ☐ ☐ ☐ ☐ ☐ ☐			
	Cups of Fruits/Veggies	☐ ☐ ☐ ☐ ☐ ☐ ☐ ☐ ☐ ☐ ☐ ☐			
	Hours of Sleep	☐ ☐ ☐ ☐ ☐ ☐ ☐ ☐ ☐			

EXERCISE	Activity	Minutes	Calories Burned

Notes:
....
....
....

Rate how closely you met your goals for today

☐ ☐ ☐ ☐ ☐ ☐ ☐ ☐ ☐ ☐
10% 20% 30% 40% 50% 60% 70% 80% 90% 100%

Day 25

Day of the Week | Date:

Time: ....

	Food/Beverage	Calories	Carbs	Fat	Protein	
BREAKFAST						
	Subtotals:					

Time: ....

	Food/Beverage	Calories	Carbs	Fat	Protein	
SNACK / SMALL MEAL						
	Subtotals:					

Time: ....

	Food/Beverage	Calories	Carbs	Fat	Protein	
LUNCH						
	Subtotals:					

Time: ....

	Food/Beverage	Calories	Carbs	Fat	Protein	
SNACK / SMALL MEAL						
	Subtotals:					

Time:	Food/Beverage	Calories	Carbs	Fat	Protein	
DINNER						
	Subtotals:					

Time:	Food/Beverage	Calories	Carbs	Fat	Protein	
SNACK / SMALL MEAL						
	Subtotals:					

DAILY TOTALS	Food/Beverage					
	Cups of Water	☐☐☐☐☐☐☐☐☐☐☐☐☐☐				
	Cups of Fruits/Veggies	☐☐☐☐☐☐☐☐☐☐☐☐				
	Hours of Sleep	☐☐☐☐☐☐☐☐☐				

	Activity	Minutes	Calories Burned
EXERCISE			

Notes:

....

....

....

Rate how closely you met your goals for today

☐ ☐ ☐ ☐ ☐ ☐ ☐ ☐ ☐ ☐
10% 20% 30% 40% 50% 60% 70% 80% 90% 100%

Day 26

Day of the Week | Date:

Time: ....

	Food/Beverage	Calories	Carbs	Fat	Protein	
BREAKFAST						
	Subtotals:					

Time: ....

	Food/Beverage	Calories	Carbs	Fat	Protein	
SNACK / SMALL MEAL						
	Subtotals:					

Time: ....

	Food/Beverage	Calories	Carbs	Fat	Protein	
LUNCH						
	Subtotals:					

Time: ....

	Food/Beverage	Calories	Carbs	Fat	Protein	
SNACK / SMALL MEAL						
	Subtotals:					

Time:	Food/Beverage	Calories	Carbs	Fat	Protein
DINNER					
	Subtotals:				

Time:					
SNACK / SMALL MEAL					
	Subtotals:				

DAILY TOTALS	Food/Beverage				
	Cups of Water	☐☐☐☐☐☐☐☐☐☐☐☐☐☐			
	Cups of Fruits/Veggies	☐☐☐☐☐☐☐☐☐☐☐☐			
	Hours of Sleep	☐☐☐☐☐☐☐☐☐			

	Activity	Minutes	Calories Burned
EXERCISE			

Notes: ....
....
....

Rate how closely you met your goals for today

☐ ☐ ☐ ☐ ☐ ☐ ☐ ☐ ☐ ☐
10% 20% 30% 40% 50% 60% 70% 80% 90% 100%

Day 27

Day of the Week | Date:

Time:	Food/Beverage	Calories	Carbs	Fat	Protein	
BREAKFAST						
	Subtotals:					

Time:						
SNACK / SMALL MEAL						
	Subtotals:					

Time:						
LUNCH						
	Subtotals:					

Time:						
SNACK / SMALL MEAL						
	Subtotals:					

Time:	Food/Beverage	Calories	Carbs	Fat	Protein
DINNER					
	Subtotals:				

Time:					
SNACK / SMALL MEAL					
	Subtotals:				

DAILY TOTALS	Food/Beverage				
	Cups of Water	☐☐☐☐☐☐☐☐☐☐☐☐☐☐			
	Cups of Fruits/Veggies	☐☐☐☐☐☐☐☐☐☐☐☐			
	Hours of Sleep	☐☐☐☐☐☐☐☐☐☐			

EXERCISE	Activity	Minutes	Calories Burned

Notes: ....

....

....

Rate how closely you met your goals for today

☐	☐	☐	☐	☐	☐	☐	☐	☐	☐
10%	20%	30%	40%	50%	60%	70%	80%	90%	100%

Day 28

Day of the Week | Date:

Time: ....

	Food/Beverage	Calories	Carbs	Fat	Protein
BREAKFAST					
	Subtotals:				

Time: ....

	Food/Beverage	Calories	Carbs	Fat	Protein
SNACK / SMALL MEAL					
	Subtotals:				

Time: ....

	Food/Beverage	Calories	Carbs	Fat	Protein
LUNCH					
	Subtotals:				

Time: ....

	Food/Beverage	Calories	Carbs	Fat	Protein
SNACK / SMALL MEAL					
	Subtotals:				

Time:	Food/Beverage	Calories	Carbs	Fat	Protein
DINNER					
	Subtotals:				

Time:					
SNACK / SMALL MEAL					
	Subtotals:				

DAILY TOTALS	Food/Beverage				
	Cups of Water	☐☐☐☐☐☐☐☐☐☐☐☐☐☐			
	Cups of Fruits/Veggies	☐☐☐☐☐☐☐☐☐☐☐			
	Hours of Sleep	☐☐☐☐☐☐☐☐☐			

EXERCISE	Activity	Minutes	Calories Burned

Notes: ....
....
....

Rate how closely you met your goals for today

☐ ☐ ☐ ☐ ☐ ☐ ☐ ☐ ☐ ☐
10% 20% 30% 40% 50% 60% 70% 80% 90% 100%

28-DAY CHECK-IN

Notes

Date:

_____

_____

_____

_____

_____

_____

_____

_____

_____

_____

_____

Current Stats

	Current	Goal
Weight		
Upper Arms		
Chest		
Waist		
Hips		
Thighs		
Calves		

Achieving My Goals

10%	20%	30%	40%	50%	60%	70%	80%	90%	100%

My Plan

Week 5 | Dates:

Meal Planner

	Breakfast	Lunch	Dinner	Snacks
MONDAY				

	Breakfast	Lunch	Dinner	Snacks
TUESDAY				

	Breakfast	Lunch	Dinner	Snacks
WEDNESDAY				

	Breakfast	Lunch	Dinner	Snacks
THURSDAY				

	Breakfast	Lunch	Dinner	Snacks
FRIDAY				
SATURDAY				
SUNDAY				

Notes:

_____

_____

_____

_____

Day 29

Day of the Week | Date:

Time: ....

	Food/Beverage	Calories	Carbs	Fat	Protein
BREAKFAST					
	Subtotals:				

Time: ....

SNACK / SMALL MEAL					
	Subtotals:				

Time: ....

LUNCH					
	Subtotals:				

Time: ....

SNACK / SMALL MEAL					
	Subtotals:				

Time: _____	Food/Beverage	Calories	Carbs	Fat	Protein
DINNER					
	Subtotals:				

Time: _____					
SNACK / SMALL MEAL					
	Subtotals:				

DAILY TOTALS	Food/Beverage				
	Cups of Water	☐☐☐☐☐☐☐☐☐☐☐☐☐☐			
	Cups of Fruits/Veggies	☐☐☐☐☐☐☐☐☐☐☐☐			
	Hours of Sleep	☐☐☐☐☐☐☐☐☐			

	Activity	Minutes	Calories Burned
EXERCISE			

Notes: _____

_____

_____

Rate how closely you met your goals for today

☐ ☐ ☐ ☐ ☐ ☐ ☐ ☐ ☐ ☐
10% 20% 30% 40% 50% 60% 70% 80% 90% 100%

Day 30

Day of the Week | Date:

Time: _____

	Food/Beverage	Calories	Carbs	Fat	Protein	
BREAKFAST						
	Subtotals:					

Time: _____

	Food/Beverage	Calories	Carbs	Fat	Protein	
SNACK / SMALL MEAL						
	Subtotals:					

Time: _____

	Food/Beverage	Calories	Carbs	Fat	Protein	
LUNCH						
	Subtotals:					

Time: _____

	Food/Beverage	Calories	Carbs	Fat	Protein	
SNACK / SMALL MEAL						
	Subtotals:					

Time:	Food/Beverage	Calories	Carbs	Fat	Protein
DINNER					
	Subtotals:				

Time:					
SNACK / SMALL MEAL					
	Subtotals:				

DAILY TOTALS			
	Food/Beverage		
	Cups of Water	☐☐☐☐☐☐☐☐☐☐☐☐☐☐☐	
	Cups of Fruits/Veggies	☐☐☐☐☐☐☐☐☐☐☐☐	
	Hours of Sleep	☐☐☐☐☐☐☐☐☐☐	

	Activity	Minutes	Calories Burned
EXERCISE			

Notes: ....
....
....

Rate how closely you met your goals for today

☐ ☐ ☐ ☐ ☐ ☐ ☐ ☐ ☐ ☐
10% 20% 30% 40% 50% 60% 70% 80% 90% 100%

Day 31

Time: ....

	Food/Beverage	Calories	Carbs	Fat	Protein
BREAKFAST					
	Subtotals:				

Time: ....

	Food/Beverage	Calories	Carbs	Fat	Protein
SNACK / SMALL MEAL					
	Subtotals:				

Time: ....

	Food/Beverage	Calories	Carbs	Fat	Protein
LUNCH					
	Subtotals:				

Time: ....

	Food/Beverage	Calories	Carbs	Fat	Protein
SNACK / SMALL MEAL					
	Subtotals:				

Time: _____	Food/Beverage	Calories	Carbs	Fat	Protein	
DINNER						
	Subtotals:					

Time: _____	Food/Beverage	Calories	Carbs	Fat	Protein	
SNACK / SMALL MEAL						
	Subtotals:					

DAILY TOTALS						
	Food/Beverage					
	Cups of Water	☐☐☐☐☐☐☐☐☐☐☐☐☐☐				
	Cups of Fruits/Veggies	☐☐☐☐☐☐☐☐☐☐☐				
	Hours of Sleep	☐☐☐☐☐☐☐☐☐				

EXERCISE	Activity	Minutes	Calories Burned

Notes: ....

....

....

Rate how closely you met your goals for today

☐ ☐ ☐ ☐ ☐ ☐ ☐ ☐ ☐ ☐
10% 20% 30% 40% 50% 60% 70% 80% 90% 100%

Day 32

Day of the Week | Date:

Time: ....

	Food/Beverage	Calories	Carbs	Fat	Protein
BREAKFAST					
	Subtotals:				

Time: ....

	Food/Beverage	Calories	Carbs	Fat	Protein
SNACK / SMALL MEAL					
	Subtotals:				

Time: ....

	Food/Beverage	Calories	Carbs	Fat	Protein
LUNCH					
	Subtotals:				

Time: ....

	Food/Beverage	Calories	Carbs	Fat	Protein
SNACK / SMALL MEAL					
	Subtotals:				

Time:	Food/Beverage	Calories	Carbs	Fat	Protein
DINNER					
	Subtotals:				

Time:					
SNACK / SMALL MEAL					
	Subtotals:				

DAILY TOTALS				
Food/Beverage				
Cups of Water	☐☐☐☐☐☐☐☐☐☐☐☐☐☐			
Cups of Fruits/Veggies	☐☐☐☐☐☐☐☐☐☐☐			
Hours of Sleep	☐☐☐☐☐☐☐☐☐			

	Activity	Minutes	Calories Burned
EXERCISE			

Notes: ....
....
....

Rate how closely you met your goals for today

☐ ☐ ☐ ☐ ☐ ☐ ☐ ☐ ☐ ☐
10% 20% 30% 40% 50% 60% 70% 80% 90% 100%

Day 33

Day of the Week | Date:

Time: ....   Food/Beverage   Calories   Carbs   Fat   Protein

BREAKFAST		Calories	Carbs	Fat	Protein	
	Subtotals:					

Time: ....

SNACK / SMALL MEAL						
	Subtotals:					

Time: ....

LUNCH						
	Subtotals:					

Time: ....

SNACK / SMALL MEAL						
	Subtotals:					

Time:	Food/Beverage	Calories	Carbs	Fat	Protein	
DINNER						
	Subtotals:					

Time:						
SNACK / SMALL MEAL						
	Subtotals:					

DAILY TOTALS	Food/Beverage				
	Cups of Water	☐☐☐☐☐☐☐☐☐☐☐☐☐☐☐			
	Cups of Fruits/Veggies	☐☐☐☐☐☐☐☐☐☐☐☐			
	Hours of Sleep	☐☐☐☐☐☐☐☐☐			

EXERCISE	Activity	Minutes	Calories Burned

Notes:

....

....

....

Rate how closely you met your goals for today

☐ ☐ ☐ ☐ ☐ ☐ ☐ ☐ ☐ ☐
10% 20% 30% 40% 50% 60% 70% 80% 90% 100%

Day 34

Day of the Week | Date:

Time: ....   Food/Beverage   Calories   Carbs   Fat   Protein

BREAKFAST		Calories	Carbs	Fat	Protein
	Subtotals:				

Time: ....

SNACK / SMALL MEAL					
	Subtotals:				

Time: ....

LUNCH					
	Subtotals:				

Time: ....

SNACK / SMALL MEAL					
	Subtotals:				

Time: _____	Food/Beverage	Calories	Carbs	Fat	Protein
DINNER					
	Subtotals:				

Time: _____					
SNACK / SMALL MEAL					
	Subtotals:				

DAILY TOTALS					
	Food/Beverage				
	Cups of Water	☐☐☐☐☐☐☐☐☐☐☐☐☐☐			
	Cups of Fruits/Veggies	☐☐☐☐☐☐☐☐☐☐☐☐			
	Hours of Sleep	☐☐☐☐☐☐☐☐☐☐			

	Activity	Minutes	Calories Burned
EXERCISE			

Notes: ....

....

....

Rate how closely you met your goals for today

☐ ☐ ☐ ☐ ☐ ☐ ☐ ☐ ☐ ☐
10% 20% 30% 40% 50% 60% 70% 80% 90% 100%

Day 35

Day of the Week | Date:

Time: ....

	Food/Beverage	Calories	Carbs	Fat	Protein
BREAKFAST					
	Subtotals:				

Time: ....

	Food/Beverage	Calories	Carbs	Fat	Protein
SNACK / SMALL MEAL					
	Subtotals:				

Time: ....

	Food/Beverage	Calories	Carbs	Fat	Protein
LUNCH					
	Subtotals:				

Time: ....

	Food/Beverage	Calories	Carbs	Fat	Protein
SNACK / SMALL MEAL					
	Subtotals:				

Time:	Food/Beverage	Calories	Carbs	Fat	Protein
DINNER					
	Subtotals:				

Time:	Food/Beverage	Calories	Carbs	Fat	Protein
SNACK / SMALL MEAL					
	Subtotals:				

DAILY TOTALS					
	Food/Beverage				
	Cups of Water	☐☐☐☐☐☐☐☐☐☐☐☐☐☐			
	Cups of Fruits / Veggies	☐☐☐☐☐☐☐☐☐☐☐☐			
	Hours of Sleep	☐☐☐☐☐☐☐☐☐☐			

	Activity	Minutes	Calories Burned
EXERCISE			

Notes: ....
....
....

Rate how closely you met your goals for today

☐ ☐ ☐ ☐ ☐ ☐ ☐ ☐ ☐ ☐
10% 20% 30% 40% 50% 60% 70% 80% 90% 100%

Meal Planner

	Breakfast	Lunch	Dinner	Snacks
MONDAY				
TUESDAY				
WEDNESDAY				
THURSDAY				

	Breakfast	Lunch	Dinner	Snacks
FRIDAY				

	Breakfast	Lunch	Dinner	Snacks
SATURDAY				

	Breakfast	Lunch	Dinner	Snacks
SUNDAY				

Notes:

Day 36

Day of the Week | Date:

Time: _____

	Food/Beverage	Calories	Carbs	Fat	Protein
BREAKFAST					
	Subtotals:				

Time: _____

	Food/Beverage	Calories	Carbs	Fat	Protein
SNACK / SMALL MEAL					
	Subtotals:				

Time: _____

	Food/Beverage	Calories	Carbs	Fat	Protein
LUNCH					
	Subtotals:				

Time: _____

	Food/Beverage	Calories	Carbs	Fat	Protein
SNACK / SMALL MEAL					
	Subtotals:				

Time:	Food/Beverage	Calories	Carbs	Fat	Protein
DINNER					
	Subtotals:				

Time:					
SNACK / SMALL MEAL					
	Subtotals:				

DAILY TOTALS	Food/Beverage				
	Cups of Water	☐☐☐☐☐☐☐☐☐☐☐☐☐☐			
	Cups of Fruits / Veggies	☐☐☐☐☐☐☐☐☐☐☐☐			
	Hours of Sleep	☐☐☐☐☐☐☐☐☐☐			

	Activity	Minutes	Calories Burned
EXERCISE			

Notes:
....
....
....

Rate how closely you met your goals for today

☐ ☐ ☐ ☐ ☐ ☐ ☐ ☐ ☐ ☐
10% 20% 30% 40% 50% 60% 70% 80% 90% 100%

Day 37

Time: ....

	Food/Beverage	Calories	Carbs	Fat	Protein
BREAKFAST					
	Subtotals:				

Time: ....

	Food/Beverage	Calories	Carbs	Fat	Protein
SNACK / SMALL MEAL					
	Subtotals:				

Time: ....

	Food/Beverage	Calories	Carbs	Fat	Protein
LUNCH					
	Subtotals:				

Time: ....

	Food/Beverage	Calories	Carbs	Fat	Protein
SNACK / SMALL MEAL					
	Subtotals:				

Time: _____	Food/Beverage	Calories	Carbs	Fat	Protein
DINNER					
	Subtotals:				

Time: _____		Calories	Carbs	Fat	Protein
SNACK / SMALL MEAL					
	Subtotals:				

DAILY TOTALS					
	Food/Beverage				
	Cups of Water	☐☐☐☐☐☐☐☐☐☐☐☐☐☐			
	Cups of Fruits/Veggies	☐☐☐☐☐☐☐☐☐☐☐			
	Hours of Sleep	☐☐☐☐☐☐☐☐☐			

EXERCISE	Activity	Minutes	Calories Burned

Notes: ....

....

....

Rate how closely you met your goals for today

☐ ☐ ☐ ☐ ☐ ☐ ☐ ☐ ☐ ☐
10% 20% 30% 40% 50% 60% 70% 80% 90% 100%

Day 38

Day of the Week | Date:

Time: _____	Food/Beverage	Calories	Carbs	Fat	Protein
BREAKFAST					
Subtotals:					

Time: _____	Food/Beverage	Calories	Carbs	Fat	Protein
SNACK / SMALL MEAL					
Subtotals:					

Time: _____	Food/Beverage	Calories	Carbs	Fat	Protein
LUNCH					
Subtotals:					

Time: _____	Food/Beverage	Calories	Carbs	Fat	Protein
SNACK / SMALL MEAL					
Subtotals:					

Time:	Food/Beverage	Calories	Carbs	Fat	Protein
DINNER					
	Subtotals:				

Time:					
SNACK / SMALL MEAL					
	Subtotals:				

DAILY TOTALS					
	Food/Beverage				
	Cups of Water	☐☐☐☐☐☐☐☐☐☐☐☐☐☐☐			
	Cups of Fruits/Veggies	☐☐☐☐☐☐☐☐☐☐☐☐☐			
	Hours of Sleep	☐☐☐☐☐☐☐☐☐☐			

	Activity	Minutes	Calories Burned
EXERCISE			

Notes:
....
....
....

Rate how closely you met your goals for today

☐ ☐ ☐ ☐ ☐ ☐ ☐ ☐ ☐ ☐
10% 20% 30% 40% 50% 60% 70% 80% 90% 100%

Day 39

Time:	Food/Beverage	Calories	Carbs	Fat	Protein
BREAKFAST					
	Subtotals:				

Time:	Food/Beverage	Calories	Carbs	Fat	Protein
SNACK / SMALL MEAL					
	Subtotals:				

Time:	Food/Beverage	Calories	Carbs	Fat	Protein
LUNCH					
	Subtotals:				

Time:	Food/Beverage	Calories	Carbs	Fat	Protein
SNACK / SMALL MEAL					
	Subtotals:				

Time:	Food/Beverage	Calories	Carbs	Fat	Protein
DINNER					
	Subtotals:				

Time:					
SNACK / SMALL MEAL					
	Subtotals:				

DAILY TOTALS			
Food/Beverage			
Cups of Water	☐☐☐☐☐☐☐☐☐☐☐☐☐☐☐		
Cups of Fruits/Veggies	☐☐☐☐☐☐☐☐☐☐☐☐		
Hours of Sleep	☐☐☐☐☐☐☐☐☐		

	Activity	Minutes	Calories Burned
EXERCISE			

Notes: ....
....
....

Rate how closely you met your goals for today

☐ ☐ ☐ ☐ ☐ ☐ ☐ ☐ ☐ ☐
10% 20% 30% 40% 50% 60% 70% 80% 90% 100%

Day 40

Day of the Week | Date:

Time: ....

	Food/Beverage	Calories	Carbs	Fat	Protein
BREAKFAST					
	Subtotals:				

Time: ....

	Food/Beverage	Calories	Carbs	Fat	Protein
SNACK / SMALL MEAL					
	Subtotals:				

Time: ....

	Food/Beverage	Calories	Carbs	Fat	Protein
LUNCH					
	Subtotals:				

Time: ....

	Food/Beverage	Calories	Carbs	Fat	Protein
SNACK / SMALL MEAL					
	Subtotals:				

Time:	Food/Beverage	Calories	Carbs	Fat	Protein	
DINNER						
	Subtotals:					

Time:						
SNACK / SMALL MEAL						
	Subtotals:					

DAILY TOTALS						
	Food/Beverage					
	Cups of Water	☐☐☐☐☐☐☐☐☐☐☐☐☐☐☐				
	Cups of Fruits/Veggies	☐☐☐☐☐☐☐☐☐☐☐☐				
	Hours of Sleep	☐☐☐☐☐☐☐☐☐				

	Activity	Minutes	Calories Burned
EXERCISE			

Notes:
....
....
....

Rate how closely you met your goals for today

☐ ☐ ☐ ☐ ☐ ☐ ☐ ☐ ☐ ☐
10% 20% 30% 40% 50% 60% 70% 80% 90% 100%

Day 41

Day of the Week | Date:

Time: ....

	Food/Beverage	Calories	Carbs	Fat	Protein
BREAKFAST					
	Subtotals:				

Time: ....

	Food/Beverage	Calories	Carbs	Fat	Protein
SNACK / SMALL MEAL					
	Subtotals:				

Time: ....

	Food/Beverage	Calories	Carbs	Fat	Protein
LUNCH					
	Subtotals:				

Time: ....

	Food/Beverage	Calories	Carbs	Fat	Protein
SNACK / SMALL MEAL					
	Subtotals:				

Time: _____	Food/Beverage	Calories	Carbs	Fat	Protein	
DINNER						
	Subtotals:					

Time: _____	Food/Beverage	Calories	Carbs	Fat	Protein	
SNACK / SMALL MEAL						
	Subtotals:					

DAILY TOTALS	Food/Beverage					
	Cups of Water	☐☐☐☐☐☐☐☐☐☐☐☐☐☐				
	Cups of Fruits/Veggies	☐☐☐☐☐☐☐☐☐☐☐☐				
	Hours of Sleep	☐☐☐☐☐☐☐☐☐				

	Activity	Minutes	Calories Burned
EXERCISE			

Notes: ....
....
....

Rate how closely you met your goals for today

☐ ☐ ☐ ☐ ☐ ☐ ☐ ☐ ☐ ☐
10% 20% 30% 40% 50% 60% 70% 80% 90% 100%

Day 42

Time: ....

	Food/Beverage	Calories	Carbs	Fat	Protein
BREAKFAST					
	Subtotals:				

Time: ....

	Food/Beverage	Calories	Carbs	Fat	Protein
SNACK / SMALL MEAL					
	Subtotals:				

Time: ....

	Food/Beverage	Calories	Carbs	Fat	Protein
LUNCH					
	Subtotals:				

Time: ....

	Food/Beverage	Calories	Carbs	Fat	Protein
SNACK / SMALL MEAL					
	Subtotals:				

Time: _____	Food/Beverage	Calories	Carbs	Fat	Protein
DINNER					
	Subtotals:				

Time: _____					
SNACK / SMALL MEAL					
	Subtotals:				

DAILY TOTALS				
Food/Beverage				
Cups of Water	☐☐☐☐☐☐☐☐☐☐☐☐☐☐			
Cups of Fruits / Veggies	☐☐☐☐☐☐☐☐☐☐☐			
Hours of Sleep	☐☐☐☐☐☐☐☐☐			

	Activity	Minutes	Calories Burned
EXERCISE			

Notes: _____

Rate how closely you met your goals for today

☐ ☐ ☐ ☐ ☐ ☐ ☐ ☐ ☐ ☐
10% 20% 30% 40% 50% 60% 70% 80% 90% 100%

Meal Planner

	Breakfast	Lunch	Dinner	Snacks
MONDAY				
TUESDAY				
WEDNESDAY				
THURSDAY				

	Breakfast	Lunch	Dinner	Snacks
FRIDAY				
SATURDAY				
SUNDAY				

Notes:

Day 43

Day of the Week | Date:

Time:	Food/Beverage	Calories	Carbs	Fat	Protein
BREAKFAST					
	Subtotals:				

Time:					
SNACK / SMALL MEAL					
	Subtotals:				

Time:					
LUNCH					
	Subtotals:				

Time:					
SNACK / SMALL MEAL					
	Subtotals:				

Time:	Food/Beverage	Calories	Carbs	Fat	Protein
DINNER					
	Subtotals:				

Time:	Food/Beverage	Calories	Carbs	Fat	Protein
SNACK / SMALL MEAL					
	Subtotals:				

DAILY TOTALS	Food/Beverage				
	Cups of Water	☐☐☐☐☐☐☐☐☐☐☐☐☐☐☐			
	Cups of Fruits/Veggies	☐☐☐☐☐☐☐☐☐☐☐☐			
	Hours of Sleep	☐☐☐☐☐☐☐☐☐			

EXERCISE	Activity	Minutes	Calories Burned

Notes: ....
....
....

Rate how closely you met your goals for today

☐ ☐ ☐ ☐ ☐ ☐ ☐ ☐ ☐ ☐
10% 20% 30% 40% 50% 60% 70% 80% 90% 100%

Day 44

Day of the Week | Date:

Time:	Food/Beverage	Calories	Carbs	Fat	Protein	
BREAKFAST						
	Subtotals:					

Time:	Food/Beverage	Calories	Carbs	Fat	Protein	
SNACK / SMALL MEAL						
	Subtotals:					

Time:	Food/Beverage	Calories	Carbs	Fat	Protein	
LUNCH						
	Subtotals:					

Time:	Food/Beverage	Calories	Carbs	Fat	Protein	
SNACK / SMALL MEAL						
	Subtotals:					

Time:	Food/Beverage	Calories	Carbs	Fat	Protein	
DINNER						
	Subtotals:					

Time:		Calories	Carbs	Fat	Protein	
SNACK / SMALL MEAL						
	Subtotals:					

DAILY TOTALS						
	Food/Beverage					
	Cups of Water	☐☐☐☐☐☐☐☐☐☐☐☐☐☐				
	Cups of Fruits/Veggies	☐☐☐☐☐☐☐☐☐☐☐☐				
	Hours of Sleep	☐☐☐☐☐☐☐☐☐				

EXERCISE	Activity	Minutes	Calories Burned

Notes: ....

....

....

Rate how closely you met your goals for today

☐ ☐ ☐ ☐ ☐ ☐ ☐ ☐ ☐ ☐

10%　20%　30%　40%　50%　60%　70%　80%　90%　100%

Day 45

Day of the Week | Date:

Time: ....

	Food/Beverage	Calories	Carbs	Fat	Protein
BREAKFAST					
	Subtotals:				

Time: ....

SNACK / SMALL MEAL					
	Subtotals:				

Time: ....

LUNCH					
	Subtotals:				

Time: ....

SNACK / SMALL MEAL					
	Subtotals:				

Time: _____	Food/Beverage	Calories	Carbs	Fat	Protein	
DINNER						
	Subtotals:					

Time: _____	Food/Beverage	Calories	Carbs	Fat	Protein	
SNACK / SMALL MEAL						
	Subtotals:					

DAILY TOTALS						
	Food/Beverage					
	Cups of Water	☐☐☐☐☐☐☐☐☐☐☐☐☐☐				
	Cups of Fruits/Veggies	☐☐☐☐☐☐☐☐☐☐☐☐				
	Hours of Sleep	☐☐☐☐☐☐☐☐☐☐				

EXERCISE	Activity	Minutes	Calories Burned

Notes: _____

_____

Rate how closely you met your goals for today

☐ ☐ ☐ ☐ ☐ ☐ ☐ ☐ ☐ ☐
10% 20% 30% 40% 50% 60% 70% 80% 90% 100%

Day 46

Day of the Week | Date:

Time: _____	Food/Beverage	Calories	Carbs	Fat	Protein	
BREAKFAST						
	Subtotals:					

Time: _____	Food/Beverage	Calories	Carbs	Fat	Protein	
SNACK / SMALL MEAL						
	Subtotals:					

Time: _____	Food/Beverage	Calories	Carbs	Fat	Protein	
LUNCH						
	Subtotals:					

Time: _____	Food/Beverage	Calories	Carbs	Fat	Protein	
SNACK / SMALL MEAL						
	Subtotals:					

Time:	Food/Beverage	Calories	Carbs	Fat	Protein
DINNER					
	Subtotals:				

Time:		Calories	Carbs	Fat	Protein
SNACK / SMALL MEAL					
	Subtotals:				

DAILY TOTALS					
	Food/Beverage				
	Cups of Water	☐☐☐☐☐☐☐☐☐☐☐☐☐☐☐			
	Cups of Fruits/Veggies	☐☐☐☐☐☐☐☐☐☐☐☐			
	Hours of Sleep	☐☐☐☐☐☐☐☐☐			

	Activity	Minutes	Calories Burned
EXERCISE			

Notes: ....

....

....

Rate how closely you met your goals for today

☐ ☐ ☐ ☐ ☐ ☐ ☐ ☐ ☐ ☐
10% 20% 30% 40% 50% 60% 70% 80% 90% 100%

Day 47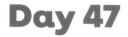

Day of the Week | Date:

Time: ....

	Food/Beverage	Calories	Carbs	Fat	Protein	
BREAKFAST						
	Subtotals:					

Time: ....

	Food/Beverage	Calories	Carbs	Fat	Protein	
SNACK / SMALL MEAL						
	Subtotals:					

Time: ....

	Food/Beverage	Calories	Carbs	Fat	Protein	
LUNCH						
	Subtotals:					

Time: ....

	Food/Beverage	Calories	Carbs	Fat	Protein	
SNACK / SMALL MEAL						
	Subtotals:					

Time: ....

	Food/Beverage	Calories	Carbs	Fat	Protein
DINNER					
	Subtotals:				

Time: ....

		Calories	Carbs	Fat	Protein
SNACK / SMALL MEAL					
	Subtotals:				

DAILY TOTALS	Food/Beverage				
	Cups of Water	☐☐☐☐☐☐☐☐☐☐☐☐☐☐			
	Cups of Fruits/Veggies	☐☐☐☐☐☐☐☐☐☐☐☐			
	Hours of Sleep	☐☐☐☐☐☐☐☐☐☐			

	Activity	Minutes	Calories Burned
EXERCISE			

Notes: ....
....
....

Rate how closely you met your goals for today

☐ ☐ ☐ ☐ ☐ ☐ ☐ ☐ ☐ ☐
10% 20% 30% 40% 50% 60% 70% 80% 90% 100%

Day 48

Day of the Week | Date:

Time:	Food/Beverage	Calories	Carbs	Fat	Protein	
BREAKFAST						
	Subtotals:					

Time:	Food/Beverage	Calories	Carbs	Fat	Protein	
SNACK / SMALL MEAL						
	Subtotals:					

Time:	Food/Beverage	Calories	Carbs	Fat	Protein	
LUNCH						
	Subtotals:					

Time:	Food/Beverage	Calories	Carbs	Fat	Protein	
SNACK / SMALL MEAL						
	Subtotals:					

Time: _____	Food/Beverage	Calories	Carbs	Fat	Protein	
DINNER						
	Subtotals:					

Time: _____	Food/Beverage	Calories	Carbs	Fat	Protein	
SNACK / SMALL MEAL						
	Subtotals:					

DAILY TOTALS	Food/Beverage					
	Cups of Water	☐☐☐☐☐☐☐☐☐☐☐☐☐				
	Cups of Fruits/Veggies	☐☐☐☐☐☐☐☐☐☐☐				
	Hours of Sleep	☐☐☐☐☐☐☐☐☐				

	Activity	Minutes	Calories Burned
EXERCISE			

Notes: ....

....

....

Rate how closely you met your goals for today

☐ ☐ ☐ ☐ ☐ ☐ ☐ ☐ ☐ ☐
10% 20% 30% 40% 50% 60% 70% 80% 90% 100%

Day 49

Time: ....

	Food/Beverage	Calories	Carbs	Fat	Protein
BREAKFAST					
	Subtotals:				

Time: ....

	Food/Beverage	Calories	Carbs	Fat	Protein
SNACK / SMALL MEAL					
	Subtotals:				

Time: ....

	Food/Beverage	Calories	Carbs	Fat	Protein
LUNCH					
	Subtotals:				

Time: ....

	Food/Beverage	Calories	Carbs	Fat	Protein
SNACK / SMALL MEAL					
	Subtotals:				

Time: _____	Food/Beverage	Calories	Carbs	Fat	Protein	
DINNER						
	Subtotals:					

Time: _____	Food/Beverage	Calories	Carbs	Fat	Protein	
SNACK / SMALL MEAL						
	Subtotals:					

DAILY TOTALS						
	Food/Beverage					
	Cups of Water	☐☐☐☐☐☐☐☐☐☐☐☐☐☐☐				
	Cups of Fruits/Veggies	☐☐☐☐☐☐☐☐☐☐☐☐				
	Hours of Sleep	☐☐☐☐☐☐☐☐☐☐				

EXERCISE	Activity	Minutes	Calories Burned

Notes: _____
_____
_____

Rate how closely you met your goals for today

☐ ☐ ☐ ☐ ☐ ☐ ☐ ☐ ☐ ☐
10% 20% 30% 40% 50% 60% 70% 80% 90% 100%

Week 8 | Dates:

Meal Planner

	Breakfast	Lunch	Dinner	Snacks
MONDAY				

	Breakfast	Lunch	Dinner	Snacks
TUESDAY				

	Breakfast	Lunch	Dinner	Snacks
WEDNESDAY				

	Breakfast	Lunch	Dinner	Snacks
THURSDAY				

	Breakfast	Lunch	Dinner	Snacks
FRIDAY				
SATURDAY				
SUNDAY				

Notes:

Day 50

Time: ....

	Food/Beverage	Calories	Carbs	Fat	Protein	
BREAKFAST						
	Subtotals:					

Time: ....

	Food/Beverage	Calories	Carbs	Fat	Protein	
SNACK / SMALL MEAL						
	Subtotals:					

Time: ....

	Food/Beverage	Calories	Carbs	Fat	Protein	
LUNCH						
	Subtotals:					

Time: ....

	Food/Beverage	Calories	Carbs	Fat	Protein	
SNACK / SMALL MEAL						
	Subtotals:					

Time:	Food/Beverage	Calories	Carbs	Fat	Protein
DINNER					
	Subtotals:				

Time:	Food/Beverage	Calories	Carbs	Fat	Protein
SNACK / SMALL MEAL					
	Subtotals:				

DAILY TOTALS					
	Food/Beverage				
	Cups of Water	☐☐☐☐☐☐☐☐☐☐☐☐☐☐			
	Cups of Fruits/Veggies	☐☐☐☐☐☐☐☐☐☐☐☐			
	Hours of Sleep	☐☐☐☐☐☐☐☐☐			

EXERCISE	Activity	Minutes	Calories Burned

Notes: ....

....

....

Rate how closely you met your goals for today

☐ ☐ ☐ ☐ ☐ ☐ ☐ ☐ ☐ ☐
10% 20% 30% 40% 50% 60% 70% 80% 90% 100%

Day 51

Day of the Week | Date:

Time: _____

	Food/Beverage	Calories	Carbs	Fat	Protein	
BREAKFAST						
	Subtotals:					

Time: _____

	Food/Beverage	Calories	Carbs	Fat	Protein	
SNACK / SMALL MEAL						
	Subtotals:					

Time: _____

	Food/Beverage	Calories	Carbs	Fat	Protein	
LUNCH						
	Subtotals:					

Time: _____

	Food/Beverage	Calories	Carbs	Fat	Protein	
SNACK / SMALL MEAL						
	Subtotals:					

Time: _____	Food/Beverage	Calories	Carbs	Fat	Protein
DINNER					
	Subtotals:				

Time: _____	Food/Beverage	Calories	Carbs	Fat	Protein
SNACK / SMALL MEAL					
	Subtotals:				

DAILY TOTALS					
	Food/Beverage				
	Cups of Water	☐☐☐☐☐☐☐☐☐☐☐☐☐☐☐☐			
	Cups of Fruits/Veggies	☐☐☐☐☐☐☐☐☐☐☐☐			
	Hours of Sleep	☐☐☐☐☐☐☐☐☐			

EXERCISE	Activity	Minutes	Calories Burned

Notes: ....
....
....

Rate how closely you met your goals for today

☐ ☐ ☐ ☐ ☐ ☐ ☐ ☐ ☐ ☐
10% 20% 30% 40% 50% 60% 70% 80% 90% 100%

Day 52

Day of the Week | Date:

Time: ....

	Food/Beverage	Calories	Carbs	Fat	Protein
BREAKFAST					
	Subtotals:				

Time: ....

	Food/Beverage	Calories	Carbs	Fat	Protein
SNACK / SMALL MEAL					
	Subtotals:				

Time: ....

	Food/Beverage	Calories	Carbs	Fat	Protein
LUNCH					
	Subtotals:				

Time: ....

	Food/Beverage	Calories	Carbs	Fat	Protein
SNACK / SMALL MEAL					
	Subtotals:				

Time:	Food/Beverage	Calories	Carbs	Fat	Protein
DINNER					
	Subtotals:				

Time:					
SNACK / SMALL MEAL					
	Subtotals:				

DAILY TOTALS	Food/Beverage				
	Cups of Water	☐☐☐☐☐☐☐☐☐☐☐☐☐☐			
	Cups of Fruits/Veggies	☐☐☐☐☐☐☐☐☐☐☐☐			
	Hours of Sleep	☐☐☐☐☐☐☐☐☐			

	Activity	Minutes	Calories Burned
EXERCISE			

Notes: ....

....

....

Rate how closely you met your goals for today

☐ ☐ ☐ ☐ ☐ ☐ ☐ ☐ ☐ ☐
10% 20% 30% 40% 50% 60% 70% 80% 90% 100%

Day 53

Time: _____	Food/Beverage	Calories	Carbs	Fat	Protein
BREAKFAST					
	Subtotals:				

Time: _____					
SNACK / SMALL MEAL					
	Subtotals:				

Time: _____					
LUNCH					
	Subtotals:				

Time: _____					
SNACK / SMALL MEAL					
	Subtotals:				

Time:	Food/Beverage	Calories	Carbs	Fat	Protein
DINNER					
	Subtotals:				

Time:	Food/Beverage	Calories	Carbs	Fat	Protein
SNACK / SMALL MEAL					
	Subtotals:				

DAILY TOTALS					
	Food/Beverage				
	Cups of Water	☐☐☐☐☐☐☐☐☐☐☐☐☐☐☐			
	Cups of Fruits/Veggies	☐☐☐☐☐☐☐☐☐☐☐☐			
	Hours of Sleep	☐☐☐☐☐☐☐☐☐☐			

EXERCISE	Activity	Minutes	Calories Burned

Notes: ....

....

....

Rate how closely you met your goals for today

☐ ☐ ☐ ☐ ☐ ☐ ☐ ☐ ☐ ☐
10% 20% 30% 40% 50% 60% 70% 80% 90% 100%

Day 54

Day of the Week | Date:

Time: ....

	Food/Beverage	Calories	Carbs	Fat	Protein
BREAKFAST					
	Subtotals:				

Time: ....

	Food/Beverage	Calories	Carbs	Fat	Protein
SNACK / SMALL MEAL					
	Subtotals:				

Time: ....

	Food/Beverage	Calories	Carbs	Fat	Protein
LUNCH					
	Subtotals:				

Time: ....

	Food/Beverage	Calories	Carbs	Fat	Protein
SNACK / SMALL MEAL					
	Subtotals:				

Time: ....

	Food/Beverage	Calories	Carbs	Fat	Protein
DINNER					
	Subtotals:				

Time: ....

	Food/Beverage	Calories	Carbs	Fat	Protein
SNACK / SMALL MEAL					
	Subtotals:				

DAILY TOTALS	Food/Beverage			
	Cups of Water	☐☐☐☐☐☐☐☐☐☐☐☐☐☐		
	Cups of Fruits/Veggies	☐☐☐☐☐☐☐☐☐☐☐		
	Hours of Sleep	☐☐☐☐☐☐☐☐☐		

	Activity	Minutes	Calories Burned
EXERCISE			

Notes:
....
....
....

Rate how closely you met your goals for today

☐ ☐ ☐ ☐ ☐ ☐ ☐ ☐ ☐ ☐
10% 20% 30% 40% 50% 60% 70% 80% 90% 100%

Day 55

Day of the Week | Date:

Time:	Food/Beverage	Calories	Carbs	Fat	Protein	
BREAKFAST						
	Subtotals:					

Time:	Food/Beverage	Calories	Carbs	Fat	Protein	
SNACK / SMALL MEAL						
	Subtotals:					

Time:	Food/Beverage	Calories	Carbs	Fat	Protein	
LUNCH						
	Subtotals:					

Time:	Food/Beverage	Calories	Carbs	Fat	Protein	
SNACK / SMALL MEAL						
	Subtotals:					

Time:	Food/Beverage	Calories	Carbs	Fat	Protein
DINNER					
	Subtotals:				

Time:	Food/Beverage	Calories	Carbs	Fat	Protein
SNACK / SMALL MEAL					
	Subtotals:				

DAILY TOTALS				
Food/Beverage				
Cups of Water	☐☐☐☐☐☐☐☐☐☐☐☐☐☐			
Cups of Fruits/Veggies	☐☐☐☐☐☐☐☐☐☐☐☐			
Hours of Sleep	☐☐☐☐☐☐☐☐☐			

EXERCISE	Activity	Minutes	Calories Burned

Notes:
....
....
....

Rate how closely you met your goals for today

☐ ☐ ☐ ☐ ☐ ☐ ☐ ☐ ☐ ☐
10% 20% 30% 40% 50% 60% 70% 80% 90% 100%

Day 56

Day of the Week | Date:

Time: .... Food/Beverage Calories Carbs Fat Protein

BREAKFAST					
	Subtotals:				

Time: ....

SNACK / SMALL MEAL					
	Subtotals:				

Time: ....

LUNCH					
	Subtotals:				

Time: ....

SNACK / SMALL MEAL					
	Subtotals:				

Time:	Food/Beverage	Calories	Carbs	Fat	Protein
DINNER					
	Subtotals:				

Time:	Food/Beverage	Calories	Carbs	Fat	Protein
SNACK / SMALL MEAL					
	Subtotals:				

DAILY TOTALS					
	Food/Beverage				
	Cups of Water	☐ ☐ ☐ ☐ ☐ ☐ ☐ ☐ ☐ ☐ ☐ ☐ ☐			
	Cups of Fruits / Veggies	☐ ☐ ☐ ☐ ☐ ☐ ☐ ☐ ☐ ☐ ☐			
	Hours of Sleep	☐ ☐ ☐ ☐ ☐ ☐ ☐ ☐ ☐			

	Activity	Minutes	Calories Burned
EXERCISE			

Notes:

Rate how closely you met your goals for today

☐ ☐ ☐ ☐ ☐ ☐ ☐ ☐ ☐ ☐
10% 20% 30% 40% 50% 60% 70% 80% 90% 100%

56-DAY CHECK-IN

Notes

Date:

_____

_____

_____

_____

_____

_____

_____

_____

_____

_____

_____

_____

_____

_____

Current Stats

	Current	Goal
Weight		
Upper Arms		
Chest		
Waist		
Hips		
Thighs		
Calves		

Achieving My Goals

10%	20%	30%	40%	50%	60%	70%	80%	90%	100%

My Plan

Week 9 | Dates:

Meal Planner

	Breakfast	Lunch	Dinner	Snacks
MONDAY				
TUESDAY				
WEDNESDAY				
THURSDAY				

	Breakfast	Lunch	Dinner	Snacks
FRIDAY				
SATURDAY				
SUNDAY				

Notes:

Day 57

Day of the Week | Date:

Time:	Food/Beverage	Calories	Carbs	Fat	Protein
BREAKFAST					
	Subtotals:				

Time:	Food/Beverage	Calories	Carbs	Fat	Protein
SNACK / SMALL MEAL					
	Subtotals:				

Time:	Food/Beverage	Calories	Carbs	Fat	Protein
LUNCH					
	Subtotals:				

Time:	Food/Beverage	Calories	Carbs	Fat	Protein
SNACK / SMALL MEAL					
	Subtotals:				

Time:	Food/Beverage	Calories	Carbs	Fat	Protein
DINNER					
	Subtotals:				

Time:		Calories	Carbs	Fat	Protein
SNACK / SMALL MEAL					
	Subtotals:				

DAILY TOTALS					
	Food/Beverage				
	Cups of Water	☐☐☐☐☐☐☐☐☐☐☐☐☐☐			
	Cups of Fruits/Veggies	☐☐☐☐☐☐☐☐☐☐☐			
	Hours of Sleep	☐☐☐☐☐☐☐☐☐			

EXERCISE	Activity	Minutes	Calories Burned

Notes:
....
....
....

Rate how closely you met your goals for today

☐ ☐ ☐ ☐ ☐ ☐ ☐ ☐ ☐ ☐
10% 20% 30% 40% 50% 60% 70% 80% 90% 100%

Day 58

Day of the Week | Date:

Time: _____

	Food/Beverage	Calories	Carbs	Fat	Protein
BREAKFAST					
	Subtotals:				

Time: _____

	Food/Beverage	Calories	Carbs	Fat	Protein
SNACK / SMALL MEAL					
	Subtotals:				

Time: _____

	Food/Beverage	Calories	Carbs	Fat	Protein
LUNCH					
	Subtotals:				

Time: _____

	Food/Beverage	Calories	Carbs	Fat	Protein
SNACK / SMALL MEAL					
	Subtotals:				

Time: ....   Food/Beverage   Calories   Carbs   Fat   Protein

DINNER	Food/Beverage	Calories	Carbs	Fat	Protein
	Subtotals:				

Time: ....

SNACK / SMALL MEAL					
	Subtotals:				

DAILY TOTALS				
Food/Beverage				
Cups of Water	☐☐☐☐☐☐☐☐☐☐☐☐☐☐			
Cups of Fruits/Veggies	☐☐☐☐☐☐☐☐☐☐☐☐			
Hours of Sleep	☐☐☐☐☐☐☐☐☐☐			

EXERCISE	Activity	Minutes	Calories Burned

Notes:
....
....
....

Rate how closely you met your goals for today

☐   ☐   ☐   ☐   ☐   ☐   ☐   ☐   ☐   ☐
10%   20%   30%   40%   50%   60%   70%   80%   90%   100%

Day 59

Time: ....

	Food/Beverage	Calories	Carbs	Fat	Protein	
BREAKFAST						
	Subtotals:					

Time: ....

	Food/Beverage	Calories	Carbs	Fat	Protein	
SNACK / SMALL MEAL						
	Subtotals:					

Time: ....

	Food/Beverage	Calories	Carbs	Fat	Protein	
LUNCH						
	Subtotals:					

Time: ....

	Food/Beverage	Calories	Carbs	Fat	Protein	
SNACK / SMALL MEAL						
	Subtotals:					

Time:	Food/Beverage	Calories	Carbs	Fat	Protein
DINNER					
	Subtotals:				

Time:					
SNACK / SMALL MEAL					
	Subtotals:				

DAILY TOTALS	Food/Beverage				
	Cups of Water	☐☐☐☐☐☐☐☐☐☐☐☐☐☐			
	Cups of Fruits/Veggies	☐☐☐☐☐☐☐☐☐☐☐			
	Hours of Sleep	☐☐☐☐☐☐☐☐☐			

EXERCISE	Activity	Minutes	Calories Burned

Notes:

....

....

Rate how closely you met your goals for today

☐ ☐ ☐ ☐ ☐ ☐ ☐ ☐ ☐ ☐
10% 20% 30% 40% 50% 60% 70% 80% 90% 100%

Day 60

Day of the Week | Date:

Time: ....

	Food/Beverage	Calories	Carbs	Fat	Protein
BREAKFAST					
	Subtotals:				

Time: ....

	Food/Beverage	Calories	Carbs	Fat	Protein
SNACK / SMALL MEAL					
	Subtotals:				

Time: ....

	Food/Beverage	Calories	Carbs	Fat	Protein
LUNCH					
	Subtotals:				

Time: ....

	Food/Beverage	Calories	Carbs	Fat	Protein
SNACK / SMALL MEAL					
	Subtotals:				

Time:	Food/Beverage	Calories	Carbs	Fat	Protein
DINNER					
	Subtotals:				

Time:	Food/Beverage	Calories	Carbs	Fat	Protein
SNACK / SMALL MEAL					
	Subtotals:				

DAILY TOTALS	Food/Beverage				
	Cups of Water	☐☐☐☐☐☐☐☐☐☐☐☐☐☐			
	Cups of Fruits/Veggies	☐☐☐☐☐☐☐☐☐☐☐☐			
	Hours of Sleep	☐☐☐☐☐☐☐☐☐			

	Activity	Minutes	Calories Burned
EXERCISE			

Notes: ....

....

....

Rate how closely you met your goals for today

☐ ☐ ☐ ☐ ☐ ☐ ☐ ☐ ☐ ☐
10% 20% 30% 40% 50% 60% 70% 80% 90% 100%

Day 61

Day of the Week | Date:

	Time:	Food/Beverage	Calories	Carbs	Fat	Protein
BREAKFAST						
	Subtotals:					

	Time:	Food/Beverage	Calories	Carbs	Fat	Protein
SNACK / SMALL MEAL						
	Subtotals:					

	Time:	Food/Beverage	Calories	Carbs	Fat	Protein
LUNCH						
	Subtotals:					

	Time:	Food/Beverage	Calories	Carbs	Fat	Protein
SNACK / SMALL MEAL						
	Subtotals:					

Time:	Food/Beverage	Calories	Carbs	Fat	Protein
DINNER					
	Subtotals:				

Time:					
SNACK / SMALL MEAL					
	Subtotals:				

DAILY TOTALS					
	Food/Beverage				
	Cups of Water	☐☐☐☐☐☐☐☐☐☐☐☐☐☐☐			
	Cups of Fruits/Veggies	☐☐☐☐☐☐☐☐☐☐☐			
	Hours of Sleep	☐☐☐☐☐☐☐☐☐			

EXERCISE	Activity	Minutes	Calories Burned

Notes: ....
....
....

Rate how closely you met your goals for today

☐ ☐ ☐ ☐ ☐ ☐ ☐ ☐ ☐ ☐
10% 20% 30% 40% 50% 60% 70% 80% 90% 100%

Day 62

Day of the Week | Date:

Time: _____ Food/Beverage Calories Carbs Fat Protein

BREAKFAST

	Subtotals:				

Time: _____

SNACK / SMALL MEAL

	Subtotals:				

Time: _____

LUNCH

	Subtotals:				

Time: _____

SNACK / SMALL MEAL

	Subtotals:				

Time:	Food/Beverage	Calories	Carbs	Fat	Protein
DINNER					
	Subtotals:				

Time:	Food/Beverage	Calories	Carbs	Fat	Protein
SNACK / SMALL MEAL					
	Subtotals:				

DAILY TOTALS					
	Food/Beverage				
	Cups of Water	☐ ☐ ☐ ☐ ☐ ☐ ☐ ☐ ☐ ☐ ☐ ☐ ☐			
	Cups of Fruits / Veggies	☐ ☐ ☐ ☐ ☐ ☐ ☐ ☐ ☐ ☐ ☐			
	Hours of Sleep	☐ ☐ ☐ ☐ ☐ ☐ ☐ ☐ ☐ ☐			

EXERCISE	Activity	Minutes	Calories Burned

Notes:

Rate how closely you met your goals for today

☐ ☐ ☐ ☐ ☐ ☐ ☐ ☐ ☐ ☐
10% 20% 30% 40% 50% 60% 70% 80% 90% 100%

Day 63

Time: ....

	Food/Beverage	Calories	Carbs	Fat	Protein	
BREAKFAST						
	Subtotals:					

Time: ....

	Food/Beverage	Calories	Carbs	Fat	Protein	
SNACK / SMALL MEAL						
	Subtotals:					

Time: ....

	Food/Beverage	Calories	Carbs	Fat	Protein	
LUNCH						
	Subtotals:					

Time: ....

	Food/Beverage	Calories	Carbs	Fat	Protein	
SNACK / SMALL MEAL						
	Subtotals:					

Time:	Food/Beverage	Calories	Carbs	Fat	Protein	
DINNER						
	Subtotals:					

Time:	Food/Beverage	Calories	Carbs	Fat	Protein	
SNACK / SMALL MEAL						
	Subtotals:					

DAILY TOTALS					
	Food/Beverage				
	Cups of Water	☐☐☐☐☐☐☐☐☐☐☐☐☐☐			
	Cups of Fruits/Veggies	☐☐☐☐☐☐☐☐☐☐☐			
	Hours of Sleep	☐☐☐☐☐☐☐☐☐			

	Activity	Minutes	Calories Burned
EXERCISE			

Notes: ....

....

....

Rate how closely you met your goals for today

☐ ☐ ☐ ☐ ☐ ☐ ☐ ☐ ☐ ☐
10% 20% 30% 40% 50% 60% 70% 80% 90% 100%

Week 10 | Dates:

Meal Planner

	Breakfast	Lunch	Dinner	Snacks
MONDAY				
TUESDAY				
WEDNESDAY				
THURSDAY				

	Breakfast	Lunch	Dinner	Snacks
FRIDAY				
SATURDAY				
SUNDAY				

Notes:

_____

_____

_____

_____

_____

Day 64

Time:	Food/Beverage	Calories	Carbs	Fat	Protein
BREAKFAST					
	Subtotals:				

Time:					
SNACK / SMALL MEAL					
	Subtotals:				

Time:					
LUNCH					
	Subtotals:				

Time:					
SNACK / SMALL MEAL					
	Subtotals:				

Time:	Food/Beverage	Calories	Carbs	Fat	Protein	
DINNER						
	Subtotals:					

Time:						
SNACK / SMALL MEAL						
	Subtotals:					

DAILY TOTALS	Food/Beverage					
	Cups of Water	☐☐☐☐☐☐☐☐☐☐☐☐☐☐				
	Cups of Fruits/Veggies	☐☐☐☐☐☐☐☐☐☐☐				
	Hours of Sleep	☐☐☐☐☐☐☐☐☐				

EXERCISE	Activity	Minutes	Calories Burned

Notes: ....
....
....

Rate how closely you met your goals for today

☐ ☐ ☐ ☐ ☐ ☐ ☐ ☐ ☐ ☐
10% 20% 30% 40% 50% 60% 70% 80% 90% 100%

Day 65

Day of the Week | Date:

Time:	Food/Beverage	Calories	Carbs	Fat	Protein
BREAKFAST					
	Subtotals:				

Time:	Food/Beverage	Calories	Carbs	Fat	Protein
SNACK / SMALL MEAL					
	Subtotals:				

Time:	Food/Beverage	Calories	Carbs	Fat	Protein
LUNCH					
	Subtotals:				

Time:	Food/Beverage	Calories	Carbs	Fat	Protein
SNACK / SMALL MEAL					
	Subtotals:				

Time: _____	Food/Beverage	Calories	Carbs	Fat	Protein
DINNER					
	Subtotals:				

Time: _____					
SNACK / SMALL MEAL					
	Subtotals:				

DAILY TOTALS	Food/Beverage				
	Cups of Water	☐☐☐☐☐☐☐☐☐☐☐☐☐☐☐☐			
	Cups of Fruits / Veggies	☐☐☐☐☐☐☐☐☐☐☐☐			
	Hours of Sleep	☐☐☐☐☐☐☐☐☐☐			

EXERCISE	Activity	Minutes	Calories Burned

Notes: ....

....

....

Rate how closely you met your goals for today

☐ ☐ ☐ ☐ ☐ ☐ ☐ ☐ ☐ ☐
10% 20% 30% 40% 50% 60% 70% 80% 90% 100%

Day 66

Time:	Food/Beverage	Calories	Carbs	Fat	Protein
BREAKFAST					
	Subtotals:				

Time:					
SNACK / SMALL MEAL					
	Subtotals:				

Time:					
LUNCH					
	Subtotals:				

Time:					
SNACK / SMALL MEAL					
	Subtotals:				

Time:	Food/Beverage	Calories	Carbs	Fat	Protein	
DINNER						
	Subtotals:					

Time:	Food/Beverage	Calories	Carbs	Fat	Protein	
SNACK / SMALL MEAL						
	Subtotals:					

DAILY TOTALS						
	Food/Beverage					
	Cups of Water	☐☐☐☐☐☐☐☐☐☐☐☐☐☐				
	Cups of Fruits/Veggies	☐☐☐☐☐☐☐☐☐☐☐☐				
	Hours of Sleep	☐☐☐☐☐☐☐☐☐				

EXERCISE	Activity	Minutes	Calories Burned

Notes: ....

....

....

Rate how closely you met your goals for today

☐ ☐ ☐ ☐ ☐ ☐ ☐ ☐ ☐ ☐
10% 20% 30% 40% 50% 60% 70% 80% 90% 100%

Day 67

Day of the Week | Date:

Time: _____

	Food/Beverage	Calories	Carbs	Fat	Protein
BREAKFAST					
	Subtotals:				

Time: _____

	Food/Beverage	Calories	Carbs	Fat	Protein
SNACK / SMALL MEAL					
	Subtotals:				

Time: _____

	Food/Beverage	Calories	Carbs	Fat	Protein
LUNCH					
	Subtotals:				

Time: _____

	Food/Beverage	Calories	Carbs	Fat	Protein
SNACK / SMALL MEAL					
	Subtotals:				

Time:	Food/Beverage	Calories	Carbs	Fat	Protein	
DINNER						
	Subtotals:					

Time:	Food/Beverage	Calories	Carbs	Fat	Protein	
SNACK / SMALL MEAL						
	Subtotals:					

DAILY TOTALS					
	Food/Beverage				
	Cups of Water	☐☐☐☐☐☐☐☐☐☐☐☐☐			
	Cups of Fruits/Veggies	☐☐☐☐☐☐☐☐☐☐☐			
	Hours of Sleep	☐☐☐☐☐☐☐☐☐			

EXERCISE	Activity	Minutes	Calories Burned

Notes: ....

....

....

Rate how closely you met your goals for today

☐ ☐ ☐ ☐ ☐ ☐ ☐ ☐ ☐ ☐
10% 20% 30% 40% 50% 60% 70% 80% 90% 100%

Day 68

Day of the Week | Date:

Time:	Food/Beverage	Calories	Carbs	Fat	Protein
BREAKFAST					
	Subtotals:				

Time:	Food/Beverage	Calories	Carbs	Fat	Protein
SNACK / SMALL MEAL					
	Subtotals:				

Time:	Food/Beverage	Calories	Carbs	Fat	Protein
LUNCH					
	Subtotals:				

Time:	Food/Beverage	Calories	Carbs	Fat	Protein
SNACK / SMALL MEAL					
	Subtotals:				

Time:	Food/Beverage	Calories	Carbs	Fat	Protein
DINNER					
	Subtotals:				

Time:					
SNACK / SMALL MEAL					
	Subtotals:				

DAILY TOTALS					
	Food/Beverage				
	Cups of Water	☐☐☐☐☐☐☐☐☐☐☐☐☐☐			
	Cups of Fruits/Veggies	☐☐☐☐☐☐☐☐☐☐☐			
	Hours of Sleep	☐☐☐☐☐☐☐☐☐			

	Activity	Minutes	Calories Burned
EXERCISE			

Notes: ....

....

....

Rate how closely you met your goals for today

☐ ☐ ☐ ☐ ☐ ☐ ☐ ☐ ☐ ☐
10% 20% 30% 40% 50% 60% 70% 80% 90% 100%

Day 69

Day of the Week | Date:

Time: ....

	Food/Beverage	Calories	Carbs	Fat	Protein
BREAKFAST					
	Subtotals:				

Time: ....

	Food/Beverage	Calories	Carbs	Fat	Protein
SNACK / SMALL MEAL					
	Subtotals:				

Time: ....

	Food/Beverage	Calories	Carbs	Fat	Protein
LUNCH					
	Subtotals:				

Time: ....

	Food/Beverage	Calories	Carbs	Fat	Protein
SNACK / SMALL MEAL					
	Subtotals:				

Time:	Food/Beverage	Calories	Carbs	Fat	Protein
DINNER					
	Subtotals:				

Time:					
SNACK / SMALL MEAL					
	Subtotals:				

DAILY TOTALS	Food/Beverage				
	Cups of Water	☐☐☐☐☐☐☐☐☐☐☐☐☐☐			
	Cups of Fruits/Veggies	☐☐☐☐☐☐☐☐☐☐☐			
	Hours of Sleep	☐☐☐☐☐☐☐☐☐			

EXERCISE	Activity	Minutes	Calories Burned

Notes: ....

....

....

Rate how closely you met your goals for today

☐ ☐ ☐ ☐ ☐ ☐ ☐ ☐ ☐ ☐
10% 20% 30% 40% 50% 60% 70% 80% 90% 100%

Day 70

Day of the Week | Date:

Time:	Food/Beverage	Calories	Carbs	Fat	Protein
BREAKFAST					
	Subtotals:				

Time:	Food/Beverage	Calories	Carbs	Fat	Protein
SNACK / SMALL MEAL					
	Subtotals:				

Time:	Food/Beverage	Calories	Carbs	Fat	Protein
LUNCH					
	Subtotals:				

Time:	Food/Beverage	Calories	Carbs	Fat	Protein
SNACK / SMALL MEAL					
	Subtotals:				

Time:	Food/Beverage	Calories	Carbs	Fat	Protein
DINNER					
	Subtotals:				

Time:					
SNACK / SMALL MEAL					
	Subtotals:				

DAILY TOTALS					
	Food/Beverage				
	Cups of Water	☐☐☐☐☐☐☐☐☐☐☐☐☐☐☐			
	Cups of Fruits/Veggies	☐☐☐☐☐☐☐☐☐☐☐☐			
	Hours of Sleep	☐☐☐☐☐☐☐☐☐			

EXERCISE	Activity	Minutes	Calories Burned

Notes: ....

....

....

Rate how closely you met your goals for today

☐ ☐ ☐ ☐ ☐ ☐ ☐ ☐ ☐ ☐
10% 20% 30% 40% 50% 60% 70% 80% 90% 100%

Week 11 | Dates:
Meal Planner

	Breakfast	Lunch	Dinner	Snacks
MONDAY				
TUESDAY				
WEDNESDAY				
THURSDAY				

	Breakfast	Lunch	Dinner	Snacks
FRIDAY				
SATURDAY				
SUNDAY				

Notes:

_____

_____

_____

_____

_____

Day 71

Time: ....

	Food/Beverage	Calories	Carbs	Fat	Protein
BREAKFAST					
	Subtotals:				

Time: ....

		Calories	Carbs	Fat	Protein
SNACK / SMALL MEAL					
	Subtotals:				

Time: ....

		Calories	Carbs	Fat	Protein
LUNCH					
	Subtotals:				

Time: ....

		Calories	Carbs	Fat	Protein
SNACK / SMALL MEAL					
	Subtotals:				

Time: _____	Food/Beverage	Calories	Carbs	Fat	Protein
DINNER					
	Subtotals:				

Time: _____					
SNACK / SMALL MEAL					
	Subtotals:				

DAILY TOTALS				
	Food/Beverage			
	Cups of Water	☐☐☐☐☐☐☐☐☐☐☐☐☐☐		
	Cups of Fruits/Veggies	☐☐☐☐☐☐☐☐☐☐☐		
	Hours of Sleep	☐☐☐☐☐☐☐☐☐		

EXERCISE	Activity	Minutes	Calories Burned

Notes: _____
_____
_____

Rate how closely you met your goals for today

☐ ☐ ☐ ☐ ☐ ☐ ☐ ☐ ☐ ☐
10% 20% 30% 40% 50% 60% 70% 80% 90% 100%

Day 72

Day of the Week | Date:

Time: _____

	Food/Beverage	Calories	Carbs	Fat	Protein
BREAKFAST					
	Subtotals:				

Time: _____

	Food/Beverage	Calories	Carbs	Fat	Protein
SNACK / SMALL MEAL					
	Subtotals:				

Time: _____

	Food/Beverage	Calories	Carbs	Fat	Protein
LUNCH					
	Subtotals:				

Time: _____

	Food/Beverage	Calories	Carbs	Fat	Protein
SNACK / SMALL MEAL					
	Subtotals:				

Time: _____	Food/Beverage	Calories	Carbs	Fat	Protein
DINNER					
	Subtotals:				

Time: _____	Food/Beverage	Calories	Carbs	Fat	Protein
SNACK / SMALL MEAL					
	Subtotals:				

DAILY TOTALS	Food/Beverage				
	Cups of Water	☐☐☐☐☐☐☐☐☐☐☐☐☐☐			
	Cups of Fruits/Veggies	☐☐☐☐☐☐☐☐☐☐☐			
	Hours of Sleep	☐☐☐☐☐☐☐☐☐			

EXERCISE	Activity	Minutes	Calories Burned

Notes: _____
_____
_____

Rate how closely you met your goals for today

☐ ☐ ☐ ☐ ☐ ☐ ☐ ☐ ☐ ☐
10% 20% 30% 40% 50% 60% 70% 80% 90% 100%

Day 73

Time: ....

	Food/Beverage	Calories	Carbs	Fat	Protein
BREAKFAST					
	Subtotals:				

Time: ....

	Food/Beverage	Calories	Carbs	Fat	Protein
SNACK / SMALL MEAL					
	Subtotals:				

Time: ....

	Food/Beverage	Calories	Carbs	Fat	Protein
LUNCH					
	Subtotals:				

Time: ....

	Food/Beverage	Calories	Carbs	Fat	Protein
SNACK / SMALL MEAL					
	Subtotals:				

Time: .... Food/Beverage | Calories | Carbs | Fat | Protein

DINNER					
	Subtotals:				

Time: ....

SNACK / SMALL MEAL					
	Subtotals:				

DAILY TOTALS					
	Food/Beverage				
	Cups of Water	☐☐☐☐☐☐☐☐☐☐☐☐☐☐			
	Cups of Fruits/Veggies	☐☐☐☐☐☐☐☐☐☐☐☐			
	Hours of Sleep	☐☐☐☐☐☐☐☐☐☐			

EXERCISE	Activity	Minutes	Calories Burned

Notes: ....

....

....

Rate how closely you met your goals for today

☐ ☐ ☐ ☐ ☐ ☐ ☐ ☐ ☐ ☐
10% 20% 30% 40% 50% 60% 70% 80% 90% 100%

Day 74

Time: ....

	Food/Beverage	Calories	Carbs	Fat	Protein
BREAKFAST					
	Subtotals:				

Time: ....

	Food/Beverage	Calories	Carbs	Fat	Protein
SNACK / SMALL MEAL					
	Subtotals:				

Time: ....

	Food/Beverage	Calories	Carbs	Fat	Protein
LUNCH					
	Subtotals:				

Time: ....

	Food/Beverage	Calories	Carbs	Fat	Protein
SNACK / SMALL MEAL					
	Subtotals:				

Time: _____	Food/Beverage	Calories	Carbs	Fat	Protein
DINNER					
	Subtotals:				

Time: _____					
SNACK / SMALL MEAL					
	Subtotals:				

DAILY TOTALS					
	Food/Beverage				
	Cups of Water	☐☐☐☐☐☐☐☐☐☐☐☐☐☐			
	Cups of Fruits/Veggies	☐☐☐☐☐☐☐☐☐☐☐			
	Hours of Sleep	☐☐☐☐☐☐☐☐☐			

	Activity	Minutes	Calories Burned
EXERCISE			

Notes: ....
....
....

Rate how closely you met your goals for today

☐ ☐ ☐ ☐ ☐ ☐ ☐ ☐ ☐ ☐
10% 20% 30% 40% 50% 60% 70% 80% 90% 100%

Day 75

Day of the Week | Date:

Time:	Food/Beverage	Calories	Carbs	Fat	Protein
BREAKFAST					
	Subtotals:				

Time:	Food/Beverage	Calories	Carbs	Fat	Protein
SNACK / SMALL MEAL					
	Subtotals:				

Time:	Food/Beverage	Calories	Carbs	Fat	Protein
LUNCH					
	Subtotals:				

Time:	Food/Beverage	Calories	Carbs	Fat	Protein
SNACK / SMALL MEAL					
	Subtotals:				

Time:	Food/Beverage	Calories	Carbs	Fat	Protein	
DINNER						
	Subtotals:					

Time:		Calories	Carbs	Fat	Protein	
SNACK / SMALL MEAL						
	Subtotals:					

DAILY TOTALS	Food/Beverage					
	Cups of Water	☐☐☐☐☐☐☐☐☐☐☐☐☐☐				
	Cups of Fruits/Veggies	☐☐☐☐☐☐☐☐☐☐☐				
	Hours of Sleep	☐☐☐☐☐☐☐☐☐				

EXERCISE	Activity	Minutes	Calories Burned

Notes: ....

....

....

Rate how closely you met your goals for today

☐ ☐ ☐ ☐ ☐ ☐ ☐ ☐ ☐ ☐
10% 20% 30% 40% 50% 60% 70% 80% 90% 100%

Day 76

Day of the Week | Date:

Time:	Food/Beverage	Calories	Carbs	Fat	Protein
BREAKFAST					
	Subtotals:				

Time:	Food/Beverage	Calories	Carbs	Fat	Protein
SNACK / SMALL MEAL					
	Subtotals:				

Time:	Food/Beverage	Calories	Carbs	Fat	Protein
LUNCH					
	Subtotals:				

Time:	Food/Beverage	Calories	Carbs	Fat	Protein
SNACK / SMALL MEAL					
	Subtotals:				

Time: _____	Food/Beverage	Calories	Carbs	Fat	Protein
DINNER					
	Subtotals:				

Time: _____					
SNACK / SMALL MEAL					
	Subtotals:				

DAILY TOTALS	Food/Beverage				
	Cups of Water	☐☐☐☐☐☐☐☐☐☐☐☐☐☐			
	Cups of Fruits/Veggies	☐☐☐☐☐☐☐☐☐☐☐☐			
	Hours of Sleep	☐☐☐☐☐☐☐☐☐			

EXERCISE	Activity	Minutes	Calories Burned

Notes: ....

....

....

Rate how closely you met your goals for today

☐ ☐ ☐ ☐ ☐ ☐ ☐ ☐ ☐ ☐
10% 20% 30% 40% 50% 60% 70% 80% 90% 100%

Day 77

Time: ....

	Food/Beverage	Calories	Carbs	Fat	Protein
BREAKFAST					
	Subtotals:				

Time: ....

		Calories	Carbs	Fat	Protein
SNACK / SMALL MEAL					
	Subtotals:				

Time: ....

		Calories	Carbs	Fat	Protein
LUNCH					
	Subtotals:				

Time: ....

		Calories	Carbs	Fat	Protein
SNACK / SMALL MEAL					
	Subtotals:				

Time:	Food/Beverage	Calories	Carbs	Fat	Protein
DINNER					
	Subtotals:				

Time:	Food/Beverage	Calories	Carbs	Fat	Protein
SNACK / SMALL MEAL					
	Subtotals:				

DAILY TOTALS	Food/Beverage				
	Cups of Water	☐☐☐☐☐☐☐☐☐☐☐☐☐			
	Cups of Fruits/Veggies	☐☐☐☐☐☐☐☐☐☐☐			
	Hours of Sleep	☐☐☐☐☐☐☐☐☐			

	Activity	Minutes	Calories Burned
EXERCISE			

Notes:

Rate how closely you met your goals for today

☐ ☐ ☐ ☐ ☐ ☐ ☐ ☐ ☐ ☐
10% 20% 30% 40% 50% 60% 70% 80% 90% 100%

Week 12 | Dates:
Meal Planner

	Breakfast	Lunch	Dinner	Snacks
MONDAY				
TUESDAY				
WEDNESDAY				
THURSDAY				

	Breakfast	Lunch	Dinner	Snacks
FRIDAY				
SATURDAY				
SUNDAY				

Notes:

_____

_____

_____

_____

Day 78

Day of the Week | Date:

Time: ....

	Food/Beverage	Calories	Carbs	Fat	Protein
BREAKFAST					
	Subtotals:				

Time: ....

	Food/Beverage	Calories	Carbs	Fat	Protein
SNACK / SMALL MEAL					
	Subtotals:				

Time: ....

	Food/Beverage	Calories	Carbs	Fat	Protein
LUNCH					
	Subtotals:				

Time: ....

	Food/Beverage	Calories	Carbs	Fat	Protein
SNACK / SMALL MEAL					
	Subtotals:				

Time:	Food/Beverage	Calories	Carbs	Fat	Protein
DINNER					
	Subtotals:				

Time:	Food/Beverage	Calories	Carbs	Fat	Protein
SNACK / SMALL MEAL					
	Subtotals:				

DAILY TOTALS	Food/Beverage				
	Cups of Water	☐☐☐☐☐☐☐☐☐☐☐☐☐☐			
	Cups of Fruits/Veggies	☐☐☐☐☐☐☐☐☐☐☐☐			
	Hours of Sleep	☐☐☐☐☐☐☐☐☐☐			

EXERCISE	Activity	Minutes	Calories Burned

Notes:

Rate how closely you met your goals for today

☐ ☐ ☐ ☐ ☐ ☐ ☐ ☐ ☐ ☐
10% 20% 30% 40% 50% 60% 70% 80% 90% 100%

Day 79

Day of the Week | Date:

Time: ....

	Food/Beverage	Calories	Carbs	Fat	Protein
BREAKFAST					
	Subtotals:				

Time: ....

	Food/Beverage	Calories	Carbs	Fat	Protein
SNACK / SMALL MEAL					
	Subtotals:				

Time: ....

	Food/Beverage	Calories	Carbs	Fat	Protein
LUNCH					
	Subtotals:				

Time: ....

	Food/Beverage	Calories	Carbs	Fat	Protein
SNACK / SMALL MEAL					
	Subtotals:				

Time:	Food/Beverage	Calories	Carbs	Fat	Protein
DINNER					
	Subtotals:				

Time:	Food/Beverage	Calories	Carbs	Fat	Protein
SNACK / SMALL MEAL					
	Subtotals:				

DAILY TOTALS	Food/Beverage				
	Cups of Water	☐☐☐☐☐☐☐☐☐☐☐☐☐☐			
	Cups of Fruits/Veggies	☐☐☐☐☐☐☐☐☐☐☐☐			
	Hours of Sleep	☐☐☐☐☐☐☐☐☐			

	Activity	Minutes	Calories Burned
EXERCISE			

Notes:

....

....

....

Rate how closely you met your goals for today

☐ ☐ ☐ ☐ ☐ ☐ ☐ ☐ ☐ ☐
10% 20% 30% 40% 50% 60% 70% 80% 90% 100%

Day 80

Time: ....

	Food/Beverage	Calories	Carbs	Fat	Protein
BREAKFAST					
	Subtotals:				

Time: ....

	Food/Beverage	Calories	Carbs	Fat	Protein
SNACK / SMALL MEAL					
	Subtotals:				

Time: ....

	Food/Beverage	Calories	Carbs	Fat	Protein
LUNCH					
	Subtotals:				

Time: ....

	Food/Beverage	Calories	Carbs	Fat	Protein
SNACK / SMALL MEAL					
	Subtotals:				

Time:	Food/Beverage	Calories	Carbs	Fat	Protein
DINNER					
	Subtotals:				

Time:					
SNACK / SMALL MEAL					
	Subtotals:				

DAILY TOTALS			
Food/Beverage			
Cups of Water	☐☐☐☐☐☐☐☐☐☐☐☐☐☐		
Cups of Fruits/Veggies	☐☐☐☐☐☐☐☐☐☐☐☐		
Hours of Sleep	☐☐☐☐☐☐☐☐☐		

	Activity	Minutes	Calories Burned
EXERCISE			

Notes:

Rate how closely you met your goals for today

☐ ☐ ☐ ☐ ☐ ☐ ☐ ☐ ☐ ☐
10% 20% 30% 40% 50% 60% 70% 80% 90% 100%

Day 81

Day of the Week | Date:

Time:	Food/Beverage	Calories	Carbs	Fat	Protein
BREAKFAST					
	Subtotals:				

Time:	Food/Beverage	Calories	Carbs	Fat	Protein
SNACK / SMALL MEAL					
	Subtotals:				

Time:	Food/Beverage	Calories	Carbs	Fat	Protein
LUNCH					
	Subtotals:				

Time:	Food/Beverage	Calories	Carbs	Fat	Protein
SNACK / SMALL MEAL					
	Subtotals:				

Time: _____	Food/Beverage	Calories	Carbs	Fat	Protein	
DINNER						
	Subtotals:					

Time: _____	Food/Beverage	Calories	Carbs	Fat	Protein	
SNACK / SMALL MEAL						
	Subtotals:					

DAILY TOTALS	Food/Beverage				
	Cups of Water	☐☐☐☐☐☐☐☐☐☐☐☐☐☐			
	Cups of Fruits/Veggies	☐☐☐☐☐☐☐☐☐☐☐			
	Hours of Sleep	☐☐☐☐☐☐☐☐☐			

EXERCISE	Activity	Minutes	Calories Burned

Notes:
_____
_____
_____

Rate how closely you met your goals for today

☐ ☐ ☐ ☐ ☐ ☐ ☐ ☐ ☐ ☐
10% 20% 30% 40% 50% 60% 70% 80% 90% 100%

Day 82

Day of the Week | Date:

Time:	Food/Beverage	Calories	Carbs	Fat	Protein
BREAKFAST					
	Subtotals:				

Time:	Food/Beverage	Calories	Carbs	Fat	Protein
SNACK / SMALL MEAL					
	Subtotals:				

Time:	Food/Beverage	Calories	Carbs	Fat	Protein
LUNCH					
	Subtotals:				

Time:	Food/Beverage	Calories	Carbs	Fat	Protein
SNACK / SMALL MEAL					
	Subtotals:				

Time:	Food/Beverage	Calories	Carbs	Fat	Protein
DINNER					
	Subtotals:				

Time:					
SNACK / SMALL MEAL					
	Subtotals:				

DAILY TOTALS					
	Food/Beverage				
	Cups of Water	☐☐☐☐☐☐☐☐☐☐☐☐☐☐☐			
	Cups of Fruits/Veggies	☐☐☐☐☐☐☐☐☐☐☐☐			
	Hours of Sleep	☐☐☐☐☐☐☐☐☐			

	Activity	Minutes	Calories Burned
EXERCISE			

Notes: ....

....

....

Rate how closely you met your goals for today

☐ ☐ ☐ ☐ ☐ ☐ ☐ ☐ ☐ ☐
10% 20% 30% 40% 50% 60% 70% 80% 90% 100%

Day 83

Time: _____

	Food/Beverage	Calories	Carbs	Fat	Protein	
BREAKFAST						
	Subtotals:					

Time: _____

	Food/Beverage	Calories	Carbs	Fat	Protein	
SNACK / SMALL MEAL						
	Subtotals:					

Time: _____

	Food/Beverage	Calories	Carbs	Fat	Protein	
LUNCH						
	Subtotals:					

Time: _____

	Food/Beverage	Calories	Carbs	Fat	Protein	
SNACK / SMALL MEAL						
	Subtotals:					

Time:	Food/Beverage	Calories	Carbs	Fat	Protein
DINNER					
	Subtotals:				

Time:					
SNACK / SMALL MEAL					
	Subtotals:				

DAILY TOTALS	Food/Beverage			
	Cups of Water	☐☐☐☐☐☐☐☐☐☐☐☐☐☐	
	Cups of Fruits/Veggies	☐☐☐☐☐☐☐☐☐☐☐	
	Hours of Sleep	☐☐☐☐☐☐☐☐☐	

	Activity	Minutes	Calories Burned
EXERCISE			

Notes: ....

....

....

Rate how closely you met your goals for today

☐ ☐ ☐ ☐ ☐ ☐ ☐ ☐ ☐ ☐
10% 20% 30% 40% 50% 60% 70% 80% 90% 100%

Day 84

Day of the Week | Date:

Time: ....

	Food/Beverage	Calories	Carbs	Fat	Protein	
BREAKFAST						
	Subtotals:					

Time: ....

	Food/Beverage	Calories	Carbs	Fat	Protein	
SNACK / SMALL MEAL						
	Subtotals:					

Time: ....

	Food/Beverage	Calories	Carbs	Fat	Protein	
LUNCH						
	Subtotals:					

Time: ....

	Food/Beverage	Calories	Carbs	Fat	Protein	
SNACK / SMALL MEAL						
	Subtotals:					

Time:	Food/Beverage	Calories	Carbs	Fat	Protein
DINNER					
	Subtotals:				

Time:		Calories	Carbs	Fat	Protein
SNACK / SMALL MEAL					
	Subtotals:				

DAILY TOTALS	Food/Beverage				
	Cups of Water	☐☐☐☐☐☐☐☐☐☐☐☐☐☐			
	Cups of Fruits/Veggies	☐☐☐☐☐☐☐☐☐☐☐			
	Hours of Sleep	☐☐☐☐☐☐☐☐☐			

	Activity	Minutes	Calories Burned
EXERCISE			

Notes: ....
....
....

Rate how closely you met your goals for today

☐ ☐ ☐ ☐ ☐ ☐ ☐ ☐ ☐ ☐
10% 20% 30% 40% 50% 60% 70% 80% 90% 100%

FINAL CHECK-IN

Notes

Date:

_____

_____

_____

_____

_____

_____

_____

_____

_____

_____

_____

_____

Final Stats

	Current	Goal
Weight		
Upper Arms		
Chest		
Waist		
Hips		
Thighs		
Calves		

Achieving My Goals

10%	20%	30%	40%	50%	60%	70%	80%	90%	100%

Maintenance Plan

CPSIA information can be obtained
at www.ICGtesting.com
Printed in the USA
JSHW040334060820
7135JS00003B/5